Keto Vegan

The Vegan Ketogenic Diet for Every Day and Everybody.

The Right Way to Change Your Lifestyle, Change Your Body and Lose Weight without Losing Your Energy.

Plant Based Diet Recipes

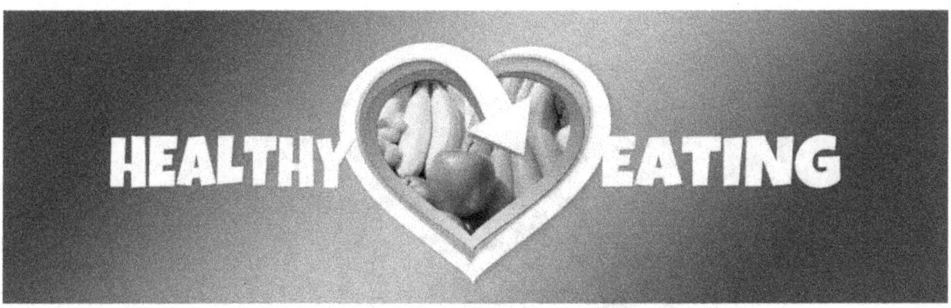

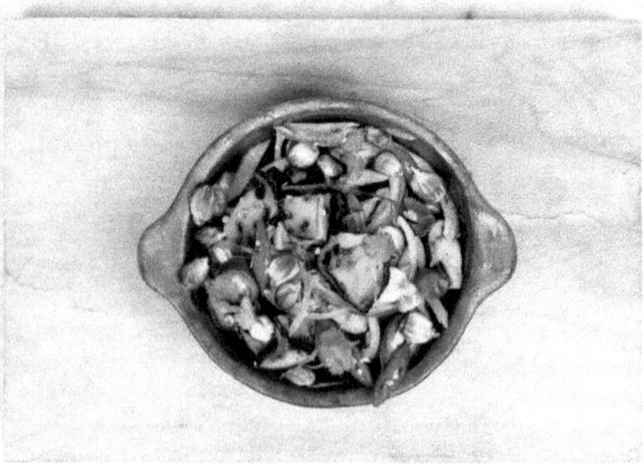

Table of Contents

Important Medical Disclaimer for Keto Clarity

The information provided by this book, *Keto Vegan: The Vegan Ketogenic Diet for Every Day and Everybody. The Right Way to Change Your Lifestyle, Change Your Body and Lose Weight without Losing Your Energy. Plant-Based Diet Recipes*, in intended only for educational and informational purposes only.

While it provides a helpful guide for people who are considering adopting a vegan keto lifestyle, you should not rely on the information we provide as a replacement or substitute for professional diagnosis, treatment, and medical advice.

We recommend that should you have any questions or concerns about your health, it is best that you consult with your medical professional or physician. All serious nutrition and medical issues must be discussed with your health care provider.

The topics discussed in this book have not been reviewed and evaluated by the FDA (Food & Drug Administration). Thus, they are not designed to prevent, diagnose, treat, or cure any disease.

Do not neglect, delay, or avoid obtaining health or medical-related advice from your healthcare professional by virtue of something that you may have learned from the book. The use of all or any of the information we provide through this book is entirely at your own risk.

Recent developments in the field of medical research may have an impact on the nutritional, health, and fitness information discussed in this book. We are giving no assurance that the information contained in this book will always reflect the latest developments or findings in the field.

We believe that the information we provide in this book is accurate at the time of writing. The content of this book is based on thorough research and our better judgment. However, just like any material, it may become obsolete over time.

The information in this book may contain some technical errors or inaccuracies and may be updated or changed without notice.

Users agree that access and use of all information in the book is at their own risk. We do not assume any liability for any information contained herein.

When in the United States and you encounter or think that you are experiencing a health or medical emergency, do not hesitate to call 911 or your healthcare professional right away.

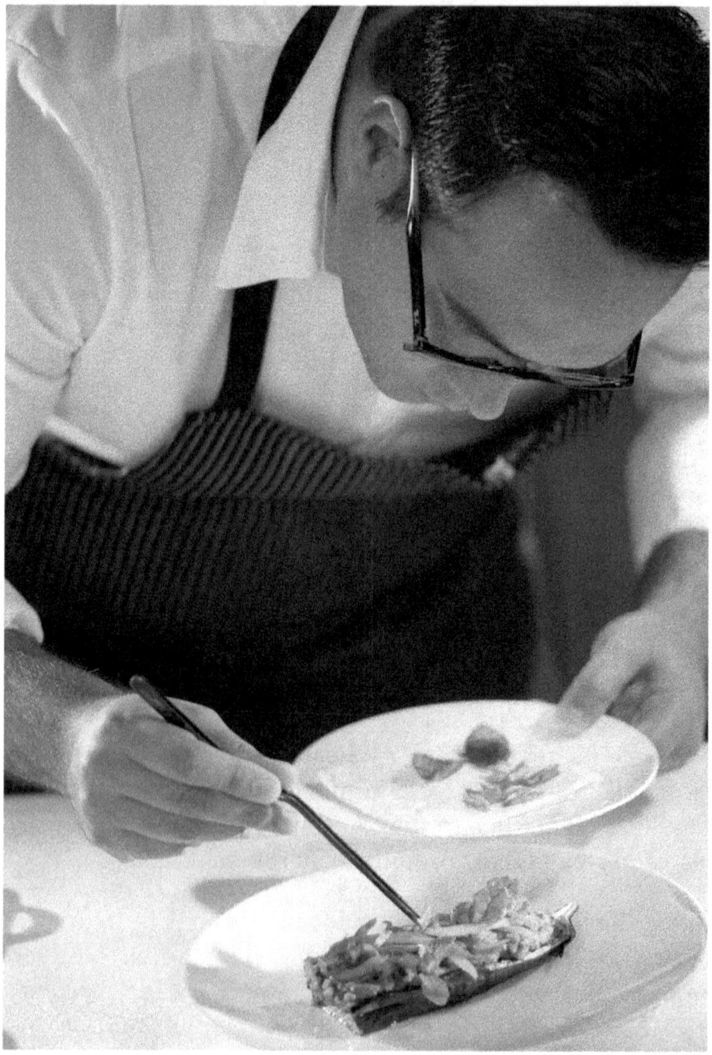

Introduction

This book contains everything you need to know about following the vegan keto diet, a combination of the ketogenic and vegan diets.

The vegan keto diet is a low-carb, high-fat regimen that focuses mainly on the consumption of unprocessed, whole, plant-based foods, and avoidance of unhealthy, highly processed, and starchy foods.

It is a combination of the vegan and keto diets that are both linked to many health benefits including weight loss, and lower risk of diabetes and heart disease.

Because of the restrictive nature of the diet, it may lack in some important nutrients that your body needs. However, this can be addressed with proper planning and supplementation with the right nutrients like vitamins B12 and D, and iron, among others.

Shifting to a vegan keto diet can be challenging. However, once you have completely adopted the lifestyle, you will start to experience a healthier and more energetic body.

Thanks for downloading this book, I hope you enjoy it!

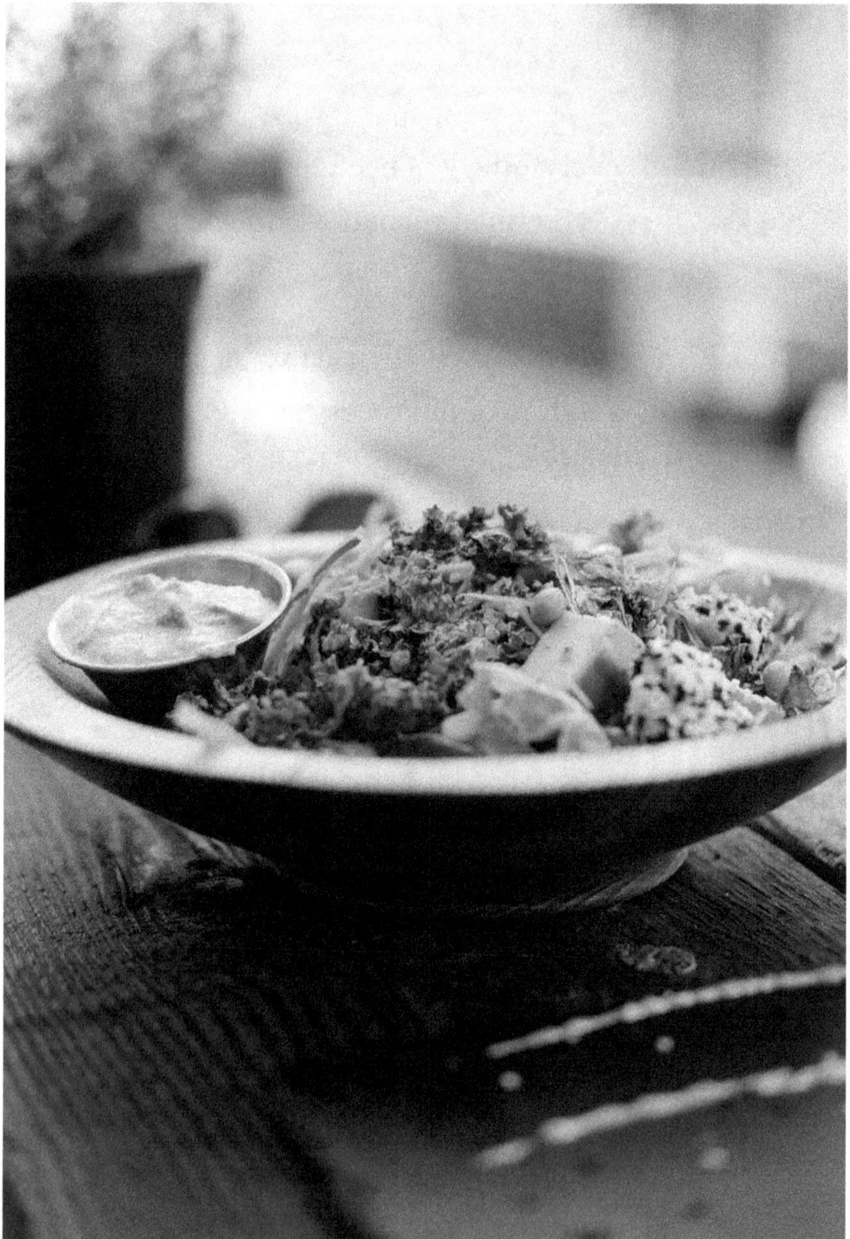

Frequently Asked Questions about the Vegan Keto Diet and Their Answers

Following are some of the most frequently asked questions about the vegan keto diet, as well as their answers:

Question: What is ketosis?

Answer: A natural process that happens in the human body, ketosis is the state of either starvation or belief that the body is starving. It is the process of using your body's fat storage as a source of fuel when the body fails to get any carbs. When the process starts, the body will shift to using fat as the energy source.

Ketosis can also happen if you eliminate carbs from your diet, and focus only on eating fats and protein. This diet will trick your body into believing that it is starving. This will then force your body to get into ketosis. In the meantime, you are giving your body a healthy food source that is nutrient-rich, helping keep it active.

Question: How does ketosis force my body to start burning fat?

Answer: When you ingest many carbs, your body converts them into glucose. Glucose then becomes your body's primary source of fuel. Your body will find no reason to turn to your fat reserves for energy or as a fuel source because of the availability of glucose. Fat will just accumulate in your body, and contribute to unnecessary weight gain.

A keto diet involves eating only food items that are low in carb content. When you limit your carb intake, your body will have no recourse but to find another energy source and this is where your fat reserves come in. The process of fat-burning for energy commences.

Question: How can ketosis help in my efforts to lose weight?

Answer: When your body is in a state of ketosis, any fat you ingest the entire day will be converted to energy. This is because your body fuels itself not from sugar from carbs. Sugar is normally the body's main source of fuel, specifically the complex and high-quality sugars. Thus, when following a carb-rich diet, your body stores most of the fat you eat, instead of using it as energy.

Consuming sugar will produce a high insulin level in your body. Insulin helps synthesize sugar and convert it into fuel for the cells in your body. However, insulin likewise suppresses your body's natural fat-burning abilities. It will lead to accumulating fat, and not fat burning.

This is a frustrating process that many people the world over try to fight on a regular basis. However, it is your body's natural defense mechanism that protects you from potential starvation.

These days, people from first world countries never get to experience starvation. Thus, they tend to eat foods that are high in carb and fat content. As a result, they store more fat in their body than necessary. This vicious cycle causes obesity.

Going to a state of ketosis helps eradicate this problem by converting the body into an efficient fat-burning machine. Because there are no carbs in your diet, your body will not have a choice but to use fat for energy. This will help you lose weight – even if you do not intend to.

Question: Is vegan keto a healthy dietary regimen?

Answer: If you are used to a diet mainly of healthy carbs such as fruits and veggies, you may think that a diet consisting mostly of fats and proteins would be quite unhealthy. You may be correct in some instances – especially if the vegan keto diet is poorly observed. You may end up consuming specific foods excessively, or not supplementing properly to maintain your overall health.

This is a real danger for people on a meat-focused ketogenic diet. Such dieters are at high risk of cramming their digestive system with excessive amounts of meat and cheese, resulting in acute cases of constipation. If you are on a vegan keto diet, however, you also need to be cautious because you are going through a very restrictive diet that may result in nutrient deficiencies.

Having said that, following the vegan keto diet for an indefinite period is safe, but only if you ensure to have a balanced diet consisting of a wide variety of food and nutrients. You should also take various supplements to compensate for the nutrients you will otherwise get from non-vegan foods. This way, you can minimize the risk of experiencing a severe case of undernourishment that will require medical intervention.

Question: What supplements must I take?

Answer: Plenty of supplements are available that can help enhance the positive effects of your vegan keto diet. Even people on a meat keto diet must also consider supplementing to make sure their body gets all the nutrients it needs to remain strong and healthy.

Following are some of the recommended supplements for keto dieters:

- Gender-specific multivitamins
- B complex vitamin
- Magnesium
- Potassium
- Vitamin D
- Fiber

Fiber is of particular importance because the diet may tend to cause constipation or intestinal slowdown. The good news is if you have been following a balanced vegan keto diet for some time, chances are, you have already been consuming fiber-rich foods. On the other hand, your fiber intake may also be very limited considering that the diet may be difficult to master, and this often results in severe nutrient deficiencies.

Question: Does the keto diet rely on calorie counting?

Answer: Majority of high carb and low-fat weight-loss diets require counting calories, and this often drives people crazy. If you are sick of counting your calorie, intake, you can rest easy because the vegan keto diet does not require calorie counting. You can consume as much food as you want – for as long as you stick to eating protein and fat-rich foods - ideally, healthy vegetables that are low in carbs. This is in addition to eating lots of fats and protein to sustain your ketosis.

Having said that, the likelihood of overeating on a keto diet is low. That is because of protein's dense nature, and protein-rich foods will occupy a lot of space in your tummy. Protein is also harder to digest, forcing your system into overdrive just to break down the nutrient to make sure that your system processes it properly. The extra work to efficiently digest protein will help keep you satiated for a longer period, averting energy dips and hunger pangs that are often associated with high sugar and carb diets.

These results to lower calorie consumption compared to a high-carb diet. In addition, you will be consuming more nutrient-rich foods. This means having less empty calories. Although your calorie consumption may not be as few as what you would get on low-fat diets, the extra calories will not matter since your body can burn the calories in a more efficient manner. Fat gives a better quality and longer-lasting fuel source for your body that can sustain you for an entire day.

Briefly, the little amount of food that you ingest in a day is converted to enough calories you can burn in a day. However, it is still crucial that you avoid excessive eating. Even if your calorie count is not restricted, overeating – even with healthy food – is a sure formula to gain weight. The key is to find the right amount of food that will make you feel full without having to eat too much. Once you find that balance, stick with eating to make sure that you will achieve your weight loss goals.

Question: How do I measure my carb intake and guard against overeating?

Answer: The most challenging aspect of the diet is ensuring that your carb intake is within the proper limits. The maximum acceptable intake ranges from 25 to 30 g of carbs for each day. The lower the level of your carb consumption, the better it is for your weight loss effort. For some people, reaching the lowest carb intake limit is extremely difficult. Thus, it is best that you find a carb intake that will be achievable for you, and then stay with it.

One way to measure, your carb consumption is to read the labels. This will give you an idea of how much you are getting for each food serving.

Question: How long does it take to get into the ketosis stage?

Answer: The shift to using fat for body fuel typically takes only a few days for most people. Limiting your carb intake to under 50 g each day, eating high fat and protein foods, and doing a regular exercise can help speed up the process. Adding more exercise is recommended as it will burn off the remaining sugar in your body, and further speed up the process. You can achieve ketosis even further if, instead of 50 g, you limit your carb consumption to less than 30 g during the first few days.

Achieving ketosis will take longer if you are obese or if you lead a sedentary life. It might take you at least a week to achieve ketosis. Thus, you will not lose weight fast. The key is to commit to regular exercise. Just a 15 to 30-minute walk each day will do you many good.

As your body starts to adopt the process, you will start to experience various changes in your body. Your mind, for one, will need to convert its energy usage to the new diet and the new ketones your body will produce. Ketones are the energy source you generate while under ketosis. Your body has been used to getting power from carbs and sugar before you shifted to a vegan keto diet. Thus, your different organs will also need to adjust to using ketones, and not carbs for energy.

This stage is called keto-adaption. Understanding the stage will help you appreciate its role in the overall keto regimen. Keto-adaption is basically the process where your body adjusts thoroughly to a ketone-based routine. Once your body reaches this stage, it will start to efficiently use the ketones for energy. Getting into the keto-adaption state often takes at least a month to achieve.

Question: Doesn't eat lots of fat make me bigger?

Answer: This is a common myth, and it is easy to see why. After all, the correlation between fat consumption and gaining weight is obvious. People know that when you eat lots of fat, your body would only store the excess fat it cannot burn. Truth is, fat is a lot more complex than what many people probably think. This is highlighted by the fact that foods have different divisions of fat.

For instance, there are unhealthy fats that are lacking in nutrients. They are simply empty calories and are called saturated fats. Consuming food high in this type of unhealthy fat will raise the levels of your unhealthy cholesterol, and increase your risk for heart disease. On the other hand, consuming unsaturated fat can reduce the levels of your cholesterol, and help improve your health.

However, eating only unsaturated fat-rich foods is not good for your body either. This is because your body needs a balanced diet to stay healthy. Healthy fats are only a part of this balanced diet. Remember the reason your body stores retain fat, and how it makes you gain weight. This link clearly demonstrates how carbs in large amounts lead to retained fat.

Fat gain happens only when you eat excessively, and your body's insulin forces your body to retain the fat in your food intake. This is because your body automatically wants to save the fat for use as an emergency source of power in times of starvation. It will store fat when you ingest a lot of food and burn fat when you do not eat at all. A high-carb diet, however, increases your chances of gaining fat because of the higher levels of insulin in your body. This makes it more difficult to eliminate the fat lingering in your body.

Surprisingly, consuming fat is not mainly to blame for weight gain. A high-fat diet can be healthy or unhealthy, and fat is not solely responsible for your unwanted pounds. Case in point is the vegan diet. Although you will rarely see an overweight vegan, it is possible. Because of the high carb diet, the minimal fat consumed is stored right away, and it does not go away. This may result in weight gain over time. By switching to a keto diet, fat will be burned more efficiently.

Question: How frequently do I eat on a vegan keto diet?

Answer: The meal schedule for a keto diet may not be the same as the eating regimen for a carb-loaded diet. Followers of the latter often eat every 2 to 5 hours, while those on keto may eat only once a day. This is because their high protein intake takes longer to digest, and it may keep them feeling full throughout the day. Deciding on the frequency of your meals needs careful planning, dividing your daily food intake into the right proportions and types of food, and then consuming everything in a span of 1 to 2 hours.

Now, you do not have to strictly follow that schedule if it does not feel comfortable for you. You can instead stick to the three meals a day routine (breakfast, lunch, and dinner) if you prefer. You can even add some healthy snacks in between.

The key is eating only when you are hungry. Avoid eating just to satisfy your craving for berries, for example. Your stomach will tell you when it is time to eat. This way, you can satisfy your hunger, and keep yourself from feeling extremely hungry at the wrong times.

If you already feel full before you have finished everything on your plate, stop eating and just put the leftovers in plastic containers. Make sure to seal and refrigerate them. Never force yourself to consume everything just to make sure nothing goes to waste. Use them when you get hungry later (though it is unlikely), or save it for the next day to save on some food money and prep time.

Hunger pangs are sometimes not real hunger and are only due to the drop in your blood sugar levels. When on a carb-heavy diet, your body will require sugar to sustain its energy. It will trigger a hunger urge even if you are still satiated.

You will not experience hunger urges when on a vegan keto diet. This is because your blood sugar levels will remain stable. Thus, you can just let your tummy tell you when it is time to eat, and you will not go wrong.

Question: why did I still gain weight even when on a keto diet?

Answer: If you gain weight on a ketogenic diet, it may be because you overeat on fatty and protein-rich foods. While most keto diet regimens do not impose caloric limits, common sense dictates that overeating is never a good idea. Your exact calorie requirements depend on your particular needs. You can do some experimentation to determine the right level for you.

In some cases, keto dieters gain a bit of weight after around 2 weeks of sticking to the diet. This often happens after losing about 5 10 15 lbs. during the first week. The initial weight loss is typically water weight, and will often balance out after 1 week. Thus, the weight gain during the 2nd or 3rd week can be quite frustrating and may throw you off the routine.

If this happens to you, do not worry. It is normal and it happens when your body starts to adjust to the diet, and its new sugar and water balance. This means you are experiencing a bit of water retention issue. The extra weight will go away in a matter of days. This temporary setback happens not only to keto diets but in most types of diet as well.

Just stick to your vegan keto routine, and experience some weight loss. If you fail to lose weight, make adjustments to your caloric intake to keep you from overeating.

Question: What are the unique demands for a vegan on a keto diet?

Answer: If you are a vegan, you can follow the demands of a keto diet without compromising anything significant. There are not any secret rules to make it more difficult to achieve ketosis.

As it is, sticking to a vegan diet is challenging enough. However, for as long as you refrain from overeating carbs, you should be able to achieve the state of ketosis, and remain there as long as you stick to the set eating pattern.

It is a good idea, however, to add more exercise to your daily routine than usual. This will help improve your protein synthesis and build your muscles. With bigger muscles, you can burn a lot more calories than fat even while resting. In short, you will be more efficient in fat-burning.

Question: How fast can I expect to lose weight?

Answer: Similar to most other weight-loss strategies, you can expect to lose around 5 to 10 lbs. for the first 2 weeks under the vegan keto diet. The rapid weight loss is often due to the loss of water, and not fat. During the early stages of the diet, you are probably burning around 3 to 4 lbs. of fat. After an initial couple of weeks, you should be able to settle down to a stable, but efficient fat-burning routine at a rate of 1 to 2 lbs. each week. The actual fat loss may vary, but not by much.

You can speed up the rate of your fat loss by adding more exercise. However, make sure to avoid too severe workouts as it may do more harm than good. It would therefore not reasonable to expect a weight loss of 3 to 5 lbs. per week. This kind of weight loss is neither sustainable nor healthy. Religiously sticking to a vegan keto diet supplemented by exercise should be enough to help you achieve your weight loss goals safely.

Question: What are the recommended exercises for a vegan keto diet?

Answer: A vegan keto diet + exercise is always a good combination. It will help improve the diet regimen's efficiency. One good thing about the diet is that practically any type of exercise will do. For instance, regular cardio exercises will not only improve your lung and heart health. They will also boost your metabolism, and upgrade your resting heart rate. This will result in improved weight loss efficiency.

Muscle-building exercises can help create a better resting state to calorie-burning ratio. This means you are able to burn more calories while in a relaxed state than before you put on additional muscles. When on keto, it is ideal to get your body in shape. This way, you will have sufficient protein to use in rebuilding your muscles, and boosting the health of your different organs. The extra fuel is necessary to sustain your organs as they adjust to a keto diet.

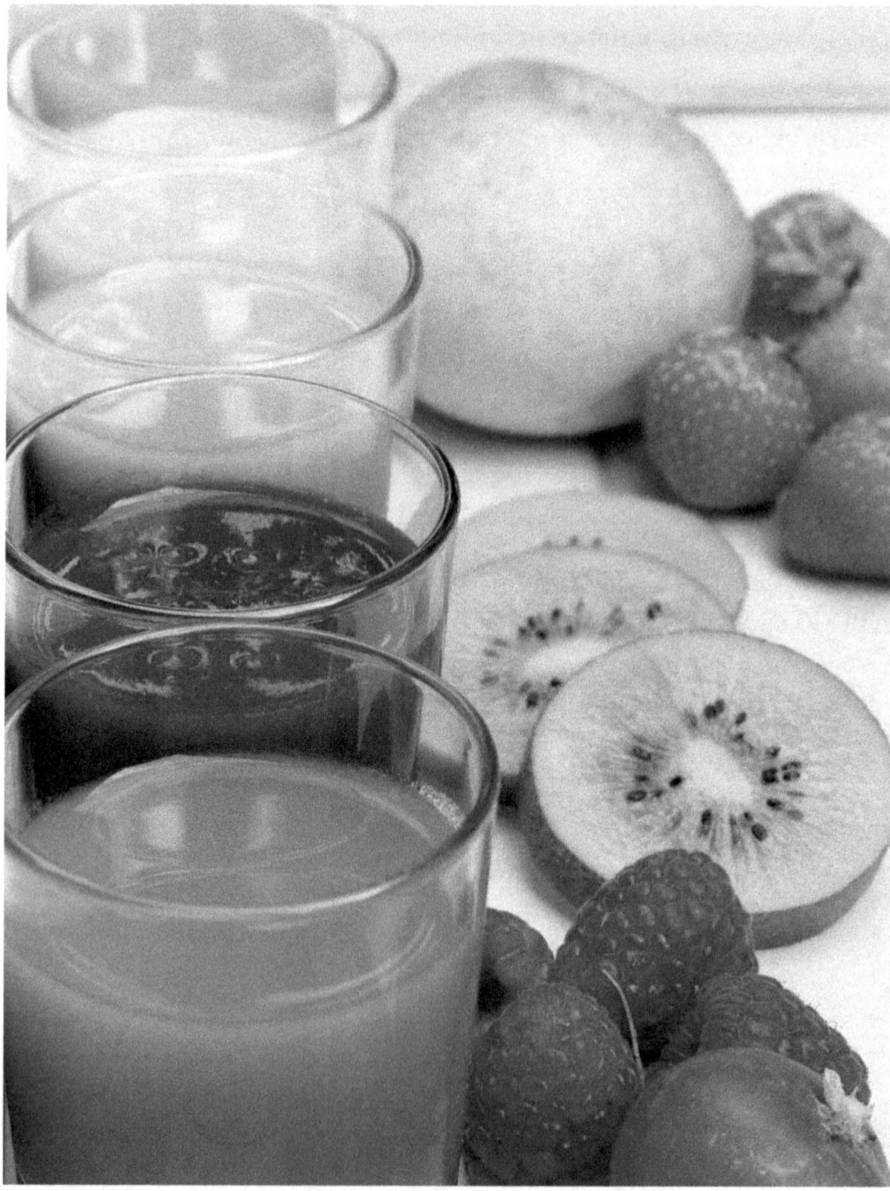

Chapter 1: How Modern Diets Make Us Fat and Sick

There has been a radical change in the diet that most people have today compared to past generations. It has become a major cause of illnesses and diseases. This is because animal-based food products contribute a big chunk of the calories people consume today.

During the past century, processed foods were practically unheard of. Today, it accounts for over 60% of the present-day diet. Sadly, natural and healthy fruits and veggies that were staples in the past, contribute no more than 5% of people's daily energy source.

Our food affects our genes, and the kind of food we eat today has led to the prevalence of various illnesses like cancer, heart disease, dementia, and obesity, among many other chronic diseases. The good news is it is possible to avoid, and even reverse the severe damage brought by a poor diet and lifestyle by eating healthy food that is rich in nutrients.

Having said that, here are some facts and information on the negative effects of poor eating habits:

Processed Foods Cause Illnesses

People need nutrients and calories from food to survive. Unfortunately, modern methods used in food manufacturing have taken away most of the nutrients from the food they process. This represents a major chunk of the calories we get from our diet.

Vitamins, minerals, as well as a wide range of other essential nutrients, provide our body with the fuel it needs to fight free radicals, neutralize carcinogens, facilitate DNA repair, and trigger an effective immune response. Decades of eating a nutrient-deficient diet have depleted our natural reserves, thus creating the perfect environment for chronic diseases to set in, and resulting in a shorter life expectancy.

Antioxidants from Food Determine Risk of Diseases and Death

The British Journal of Nutrition published a study that proved the protective effects of various antioxidant nutrients in countering all mortality causes. In particular, the proponents of the study concluded that there is enough evidence to prove that Vitamin C intake can predict all subsequent mortality causes. Previous studies have shown the same effect from consuming selenium and carotene.

The results of the studies show that the concentration of specific nutrients can be effective in predicting the risk for diseases and death. This information highlights the crucial role played by eating a natural diet that provides a wide range of nutrients that can help reduce the risk of chronic illnesses.

Children Today Develop a Preference for Junk Food at an Early Age

Many children today grow up with a diet of processed food. Thus, they develop a taste for fried, salty, and sugared foods early in their life. The instinct to eat meats, fruits, and vegetables in their natural state has been erased. Instead, their taste buds have been trained to prefer a highly processed and refined diet full of artificially manufactured chemical ingredients that are more pleasing to their taste.

According to an analysis done by the American Dietetic Association Journal, out of the 2200 calories that a typical child consumes each day, 800 is from added sugar and solid fats. These micronutrients barely provide any nutrients, and in fact, is mainly responsible for the rising child obesity problem today.

Children who develop a taste for processed and junk food early in life are a lot more likely to experience weight problems later in life. They also tend to suffer from the early onset of chronic disorders like diabetes and heart disease.

A Diet of Natural Food Can Help Reverse Disease Progression

A great majority of adults and children today consume only less than ¼ of the body's daily fruit and vegetable requirements to provide the minimum amount of protection against illnesses.

The recommendation from nutritionists is to add 5 to 10 servings of fresh veggies and leafy greens, nuts, berries, seeds, protective monounsaturated fats, and lean protein sources to your diet each day. Prepare your food minimally cooed or raw, and avoid overheating as much as possible, as this quickly takes away the nutrients.

Our body has an incredible ability to repair itself, and reverse the damaging effects of a bad diet. Health-conscious people see natural food as medicine that results in a healthier and longer life. Thus, many have started to adopt healthier lifestyles. These include the ketogenic and vegan diets, both of which are gaining in popularity today.

The Vegan Lifestyle

The vegan diet, together with Paleo, South Beach, and Keto diets, among many others, always pop up when conversation shifts to effective methods that can help you lose weight. Each diet is based on a specific philosophy that makes it work. Each one guarantees that you will lose weight in a healthy way. Some are backed up by science, while some are simply outrageous.

Let us focus on the vegan diet. What is the fuss about going vegan? In addition, more importantly, does it deliver its promised benefits?

The vegan diet involves getting rid of all animal-based food products from your daily fare. When we say all, we are talking about chicken, beef, eggs, dairy products, honey – and heck, even silk, and leather! The general rule is if an animal was used/tested/harmed in making the product, it is a no-no in a vegan diet. You cannot consume it.

For some vegans, everything boils down to ethics. Others do it because of their religion. For most people, however, switching to a vegan diet is a conscious decision to live a more compassionate (to animals) and healthier life.

As mentioned, veganism is a lifestyle, and not merely a kind of diet. Vegans do not harm, much less kill animals for sustenance.

Suddenly, a diet involves the question of morality. As humans, are we superior to animals? If so, does it give us the right to harm and eat them?

The vegan diet offers a different take on man's relationship with food. In the fast-paced world, we live in today; there is not any time to even question the source of our food. Like most other people, we simply go to the supermarket with a shopping list on hand.

We enter the store; go straight to the dry goods section, then the veggies, and on to the meat section. We simply go through the motions – without even thinking. Do we ever stop for a moment to think why this particular vegetable is good for me? Alternatively, what can this chicken do for me? Where do these food items come from? If you pause for a moment to think about these things, then you probably have a good appreciation of the stuff you put into your body on a daily basis.

This is what veganism is all about. You become not only healthier, but a better human being overall – just by practicing a vegan lifestyle. By being a vegan, you get to indirectly save a few animals, and to a certain extent, the environment as well. You also help the local farming community by patronizing their produce.

Like many other diets, the vegan lifestyle promises many great results. You will feel good overall. You will be more energetic and feel lighter.

Before you adopt any diet, weigh the pros vs. the cons. Make sure to get the clearance of your physician first, and actively monitor how your body will react to the new regimen. You may also need to take supplements like B12, as well as other nutrients that the new diet may fail to provide.

Health Benefits of a Vegan Diet

- *Richer in Some Important Nutrients* – Switching from a typical diet to vegan means eliminating all meats and animal-based products. Thus, you will be forced to rely heavily on other food sources.

  When on a whole-food diet, replacements for animal-based food items will come from fruits, veggies, whole grains, peas, beans, seeds, and nuts. These foods contribute a big chunk of a vegan diet, unlike the Western diet. Thus, they will offer a higher amount of some beneficial nutrients.

  For example, various studies prove that a vegan diet tends to contribute more antioxidants, fiber, and other beneficial plant compounds. They also have higher magnesium, folate, potassium, and A, C, and E vitamins.

However, not every vegan diet is the same. For one, when poorly planned, a vegan diet may lack in essential fatty acids, calcium, iron, zinc, or vitamin B12. Thus, it is crucial that you stay away from fast food vegan options that are nutrient-poor. You must instead build your diet around whole plants that are nutrient-rich, as well as fortified foods. Supplementing would also be a good idea.

- *Helps Get Rid of Excess Weight* – A lot of people start shifting to a plant-based diet, hoping that it will help them lose unwanted pounds. This is a valid reason. Many observational studies tend to point out that vegans are generally lower BMIs and thinner than meat-eaters.

  Various randomized controlled studies, which are considered as the ultimate standard in scientific research, say that a vegan diet is a more effective weight-loss method than many other diets.

  In one study done over an 18-week period, participants under a vegan diet lost an average of 9.3 lbs. more than those placed under a controlled diet at the conclusion of the study.

  It is worth mentioning that those on a vegan diet outdid their counterparts who were under calorie-restricted diets. This is even more impressive, given the fact that the vegan group was allowed to eat until full.

In a recent study to compare the effects of five different diets on weight loss, the conclusion was that vegan and vegetarian diets are more promising than standard Western diets and semi-vegetarian diets. Even when the vegan and vegetarian groups did not perfectly follow their diet plans, they still lost a bit more weight compared to participants under a standard Western diet.

Simply put, a vegan diet seems to have a natural tendency to lower your calorie consumption. This makes it effective for losing weight even without focusing on cutting your calorie intake.

- *Lowers Blood Sugar Levels and Improves Kidney Function* – Adopting a vegan lifestyle provides benefits for people suffering from type 2 diabetes and deteriorating kidney function. The diet helps improve insulin sensitivity, and lower blood sugar levels while reducing your risk of acquiring type 2 diabetes by as much as 50 – 75%.

  Studies also show that a vegan diet reduces the level of blood sugar in diabetics better than the diets endorsed by the American Heart Association, American Diabetes Association, and the National Cholesterol Education Program.

  According to one study, 43% of the participants placed under a vegan diet reduced their reliance on medications to lower their blood sugar levels. This is much better than the 26% in the other group that was under a diet recommended by ADA.

Other studies reported that patients with diabetes who replaced meat for plant protein in their diet tend to lower their risk of kidney function deterioration. In addition, there are several studies that showed a vegan diet might have the ability to completely relieve symptoms of systemic distal polyneuropathy, a diabetic condition that leads to sharp, burning pain.

In summary, a vegan diet may lower the risk of type 2 diabetes. It is also proven effective in lowering blood sugar levels. It may also help stop the development of further medical issues.

- *Protection Against Certain Types of Cancer* – The WHO reports that about 1/3 of all types of cancer can be stropped on their tracks by controllable factors, including your diet. Eating legumes on a regular basis, for example, may lower your risk of developing colorectal cancer by 9 to 18%.

  Research also shows that intake of at least seven servings of fresh veggies and fruits each day may reduce your risk of death from cancer by as much as 15%.

  In general, vegans consume more fruits, vegetables, and legumes than those on a non-vegan diet. This may be the reason why in a recent evaluation of 96 studies, the results showed that vegans tend to experience 15% less risk of dying from or developing cancer.

A vegan diet also includes more soy products, thus providing significant protection from breast cancer.

Avoiding some animal-based products may also aid in reducing the risk of breast, colon, and prostate cancers. This may be because a vegan diet shuns processed or smoked meats, as well as meats heated at high temperatures. Overheating is believed to cause some types of cancer.

Vegans also do not consume dairy products that, according to several studies, tend to increase the risk of developing prostate cancer. Meanwhile, evidence also points to the possibility that dairy may help lower the risk of other cancer types, including colorectal cancer. Thus, it is likely that removing dairy from your diet is not the factor that reduces a vegan's overall exposure to cancer.

Note that the studies mentioned above are observational in nature, and it is extremely difficult to identify the exact reason vegans have a reduced cancer risk. However, until the time more conclusive studies are made, it would seem like a great idea to focus on adding more fresh fruits, veggies, and legumes to your regular diet, while avoiding consumption of overcooked, smoked, and processed meats.

- *Reduced Risk of Heart Disease* – Eating fresh veggies, fruits, fiber, and legumes is associated with a reduced risk of heart disease. A well-planned vegan regimen includes these fresh food items in generous amounts.

  Based on observational studies that compared vegans to the rest of the general population, it was seen that vegans tend to benefit from a lower risk of acquiring hypertension by as much as 75%. Vegans are also less likely (by up to 42%) to die from heart disease.

  In addition, various randomized controlled studies reported that vegan diets are better at controlling blood sugar, total cholesterol, and LDL levels compared to other diets used in the studies.

  This is beneficial since lower blood pressure, as well as blood sugar and cholesterol levels, mean lower risk factors that contribute to the development of heart disease by up to 46%. In comparison to the general population, a vegan tends to eat more nuts and whole grains. Both are heart-friendly.

- *Reduced Pain Caused by Arthritis* – There are studies that prove the positive effects of vegan diets to people suffering from various types of arthritis. In one study, 40 participants suffering from arthritis were asked to either stay on their meat-loaded diet or shift to a plant-based, whole-food vegan diet for 1 ½ month. Those who partook a vegan diet showed improved energy levels, as well as better overall functioning compared to those who stayed on their diet.

In two other studies that investigated the impact of raw food, probiotic-packed vegan diet on rheumatoid arthritis symptoms, both had the same conclusion that the vegan group had significant improvements in symptoms like joint swelling, pain, and morning stiffness compared to those on a meat diet.

Veganism vs. Vegetarianism

The two lifestyles are often mistaken for one another. Truth is there are some major differences between the two, particularly in terms of nutritional intake and food choices.

A vegetarian does not eat meat but may consume eggs and dairy products. A vegan shuns all animal products. This means a vegetarian does not necessarily have to compensate for medical deficiencies by supplementation. After all, they can still have the calcium they need from milk. On the other and a vegan needs to find a plant-based alternative calcium source.

Veganism also involves an array of lifestyle choices that do not include animal-based products. Vegetarianism, meanwhile, is plain and simple, a dietary preference.

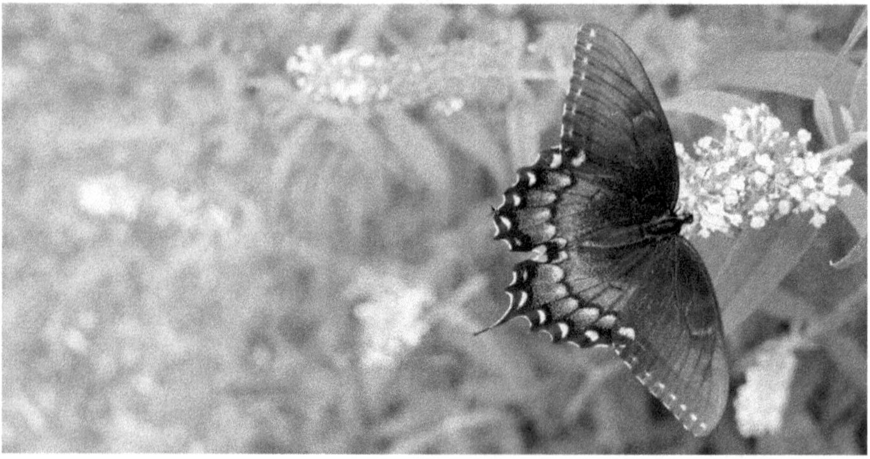

Nutrient Deficiencies to Consider before Adopting a Vegan Lifestyle

- *Vitamin B12* – The nutrient is necessary for the protection of the red blood cells and nerves. Alternative sources for vegans include nutritional yeast and B12 fortified plant-based foods.
- *Vitamin D* – Vitamin D provides protection against chronic diseases and various types of cancer. It also helps improve teeth and bone health. Alternative sources for vegans include the sun and vitamin D-fortified foods.
- *Iron* – The nutrient is useful for oxygen absorption into the blood, and distribution of oxygen to the different body cells.

Good iron sources for vegans are dark leafy greens and dried beans.

- *Omega 3 Fatty Acids* – Omega 3 is crucial for heart health, and brain and eye function. Vegans can get the nutrient from ground flaxseed, canola oil, and walnuts.
- *Calcium* – The nutrient is good for the maintenance and development of bone health. Green leafy veggies and tofu are great vegan sources.
- *Zinc* – The mineral is crucial for maintaining a healthy immune system. Good sources of zinc for vegans are legumes and whole grains.

In addition, a vegan diet may limit your calorie consumption. Thus, proper meal planning is important to make sure that you get your required amount of calories.

The Ketogenic Lifestyle

Although it has been around since the 1920s, the ketogenic lifestyle has recently been enjoying unprecedented popularity. In fact, followers of the popular Atkins or Paleo diet are shifting to a ketogenic diet by the numbers. It is easy to see why. For one, aside from helping you lose weight, keto boost your mental clarity, improve your mood, and regain or maintain your overall health and wellbeing.

So, how does the keto diet work and what should you eat to make sure you get the most out of the diet?

How Keto Diet Works

When on a keto diet, your body gets into a metabolic state known as ketosis. Once there, you will start to experience all the much talked about the health benefits of the diet.

The State of Ketosis

Our body typically relies on sugars and carbohydrates as a primary source of fuel for our daily activities. However, when you are in ketosis, your body shifts to burning fat for energy. Its reliance on sugars and carbs becomes minimal.

Getting into Ketosis

An easy way to achieve ketosis is to adopt a keto diet!

Your goal should be to eat less than 25 g of carbohydrates each day, and the rest your calorie intake must come from plenty of healthy fats, as well as a moderate amount of proteins. For now, you should not wrack your brains figuring out the exact ratios to follow. In addition, you can use simple online keto calculators to determine your macro requirements.

The key is to change your food preferences. Once you achieve that, your metabolism will follow, and your body will get into a state of ketosis – naturally.

What to Eat and Not to Eat on a Ketogenic Diet

Many people are confused when talking about a keto lifestyle. After all, it is not easy to limit your food intake to under 25 g of carbs, a moderate amount of protein, and a lot of healthy fats on a daily basis.

What to eat	Meat, seafood, low-carb veggies and leafy greens like olives, cauliflower, avocados, olive oil, coconut oil, as well as low-carb fruits
What not to eat	All grains (like corn, wheat, oats), processed vegetable oils, artificial coloring and sweeteners, legumes, high carb veggies (like regular and sweet

	potatoes), butternut squash, as well as sugary fruits like mangoes, grapes, and pineapples

Health Benefits of a Ketogenic Lifestyle

Here are the top four health benefits of following a keto lifestyle (and there are many others):

- *Effective Weight Loss* – Many studies support this claim. In one of these studies, the proponents compared a group of participants placed on a high fat, low-carb diet (similar to a ketogenic diet), with participants who were under a more conventional diet for weight loss (unlimited carbs, but calorie-restricted and very low in fat). Members of the first group lost a lot more weight compared to the second group.
- *Lower Risk of Heart Disease* - A keto diet can significantly lower your risk of acquiring heart disease. It is one of the diets of numerous physiological benefits.

  There is enough scientific evidence that shows the diet's ability to help lower the risk of heart disease. This is possible because following the keto diet can help lower high blood pressure, and improve cholesterol and triglyceride levels.

- *Significant Energy Boost* – Based on anecdotes from a lot of keto followers, the diet provides your body with lots of energy. Dieters say they feel more energetic and become more focused and clear-headed. Many say that they do not experience mid-afternoon fatigue that is common to non-keto dieters. Neither do they have to deal with forgetfulness or brain fog the entire day!

  If this is not yet convincing enough for you, you can check out a few keto diet forums online, as well as read various Reddit threads where you can see lots of real-life experiences.

- *Reduce Overeating* – Shifting to a ketogenic lifestyle can help you reduce your tendency to overeat. The diet curbs your appetite by doing a number on your hunger hormones.

  In one keto study, proponents monitored a group of participants who were placed under a diet that is similar to keto. Although the participants were allowed to eat as much as they wanted, they had lower food intake – even without their conscious attempts to do so. Many keto dieters also claim to feel fewer hunger pangs and food cravings because of the kind of food they were eating.

Starting a Keto Diet

If you are contemplating starting a keto lifestyle, you first need to focus on a few important things:

1. *Stock up your pantry with lots of nutrient-rich foods.* - Bear in mind that low-carb foods do not necessarily mean they are not good for you. Refrain from buying sodas and other low-carb but processed foods, including energy bars and drinks. Instead, focus on foods that are packed with many vitamins, minerals, and antioxidants that the body needs to achieve and maintain optimal health.

   Do not get distracted by counting calories. What is important is to make sure you eat only nutrient-dense food items.

   Action to take now: go over the contents of your refrigerator and pantry, and then get rid of every non-keto food you can find. While it may sting a bit, it will definitely help strengthen your resolve to lead a healthier lifestyle.

2. *Decide on a stress-free week to begin your keto journey.* – It would not be a good idea to start your keto diet on a busy

workweek when you are neck-deep into a big project. Your body will need about 1 week to adjust to your new diet.

During the first week under a keto diet, you may experience symptoms of keto flu. You may then need some time to adjust and get accustomed to your new healthy lifestyle. Thus, it is important to start the diet on a week when you expect a light schedule, and you can find lots of time to rest.

3. *Your diet is only one component of having a healthy lifestyle.* – Improving your overall health involves not only a change in your diet. While shifting to a healthier diet provides you with a good head start, there is a lot more that you need to do.

   For one, you need to complement your diet with regular exercise, sufficient rest every night, proper stress management, and spend quality time with people you care about and whose company you enjoy the most.

   Action to take now: Exercise or visit the gym to work out at least once for this week. Then, plan to have a date with a friend to do some fun activities.

Shifting to a keto lifestyle is a major step in your efforts to gain optimum health in the long term.

Much scientific evidence shows that lifestyle can help you feel better overall. It will improve practically every aspect of your life – from boosting your energy levels to curbing food cravings to enhancing your mood. On top of all this, you will lose weight, if weight loss is one of your goals.

Bear in mind that there is more to the keto diet than just-food. After all, it is a lifestyle, and as such, you need to combine it with healthy living. Go out in the sun to exercise, have a good laugh with friends, and get rid of your stressors. It is also a good idea to try meditation and mindfulness.

The ketogenic diet is never intended to restrict your way of living. Instead, it is designed to set you free to allow you to look great, feel great, and live your life according to your dreams!

Chapter 2: Understanding the Vegan Keto Diet

The ketogenic diet, briefly, is a high fat, low carb diet with a moderate amount of protein.

In a typical keto diet, carbohydrates are typically limited to under 50 grams each day. This is to reach and maintain the state of ketosis, the metabolic process that allows your body to burn fat, and use it for energy, instead of glucose.

The keto diet consists mainly of fat. In general, around ¾ of your daily intake is from fat sources. Thus, many dieters often rely on high-fat animal products to sustain their diet. These include meats, full fat, dairy, and butter.

If you are vegan or one who is strictly on a plant-based diet, it does not mean you cannot follow a ketogenic diet. You can continue eating your regular plant-based meals consisting of fruits, grains, and veggies while avoiding animal-based food products like poultry, meat, dairy, and eggs.

As a vegan, you can achieve ketosis by depending on plant-based products that are high in healthy fat content such as avocados, seeds, nuts, and coconut oil.

Benefits of the Vegan Keto Diet

While there have been no studies yet that focus solely on the benefits of the vegan keto diet, many health benefits are linked to ketogenic and vegan diets on their own.

For one, a vegan diet has been proven to lower your risk of exposure to various health conditions like diabetes, heart disease, and some types of cancer. According to studies, a vegan diet can lower your risk of developing hypertension by about 75%, and diabetes by as much as 78%.

In addition, vegans have the tendency to weigh less compared to meat-eaters, and if you adopt a vegan diet, you are likely to be more successful in your weight loss efforts that if you were a non-vegan. In a study published in PubMed, it was found that people on vegan diets were able to lose an average of 5 lbs. more than those who were on non-vegan diets.

Similar to the vegan diet, various research has proven that the low carb, a high fat ketogenic diet may have a significant positive impact on your health. The keto diet is mainly credited for its effectiveness in losing weight, blood sugar management, and reducing risk factors for heart disease.

In one study conducted on 58 obese teens and children, participants who were made to undergo a keto diet lost a significant amount of weight and fat mass compared to those who underwent a low-calorie diet.

The keto diet likewise raised adiponectin levels in the body. Adiponectin is a type of protein involved in the regulation of blood sugar, as well as fat metabolism.

Higher adiponectin levels are linked to better control of blood sugar, reduced inflammation, and reduced risk of diseases associated with obesity like heart disease.

The keto diet is also known to reduce factors of heart disease. These include blood pressure, LDL or bad cholesterol, and high triglycerides.

Considering that both ketogenic and vegan diets provide health benefits in similar ways, there is the reason to believe that by adopting the vegan keto diet or combining the ketogenic and vegan diets, you can enjoy the same health benefits.

Having said that, here are the top science-backed vegan keto benefits:

- *Burn Fat Efficiently, and Achieve a Healthy Weight* – A lot of people adopt the keto diet as a simple and effective way of managing their weight. Following a high fat, low-carb diet allows your body to get into a prolonged ketosis state. This makes your body to effectively burn off fat as you lose weight – even without or with minimal exercise. This is because the diet will force your body to use fat for energy, instead of carbohydrates.

There is sufficient evidence that proves the efficiency of the keto diet for losing weight. For some people, the shift in diet alone triggers considerable weight loss within a short period. It is worth mentioning that abdominal fat, which is known as very difficult to lose, seems to go away at a much faster rate in ketosis, unlike when a person is on a normal or high-carb diet.

- *Gain More Energy, and Experience Fewer Food Cravings* – When on a carb-loaded diet, your body constantly goes through a roller-coaster cycle of converting carbohydrates into glucose. This results in a rise in your blood sugar level. This is particularly the case when you eat simple carbs like sugar and processed food. While you will initially experience an energy boost, the spike will soon end, and you will feel depleted. This means you will feel hungry and start to crave for more carbs to deliver the backup energy you need.

  Keto works in a different way. Being in a state of ketosis is similar to burning logs, instead of kindling, where the logs are the fats, and kindling, the carbs. When burning carbs (kindling), the fire waxes hot for a short period, and then it will disappear fast. On the other hand, when burning fats (logs), the fire burns in a steady manner for a longer period. When in ketosis, you will experience more consistent levels of energy, without experiencing energy spikes. You will not have the same food cravings that you would tend to have when consuming carbs.

- *Lessen Symptoms of Epilepsy* – The keto diet has been known around the medical community for over 90 years now, although it has become popular on the internet only in recent years. The diet was developed during the 1920s as an attempt to imitate the biochemical process that occurs during starvation or fasting. It is seen as an effective and established therapy for medicine-resistant and hard-to-treat forms of epilepsy.

- *Provide Protection and Nourishment for the Brain* – There is growing evidence that a keto diet has neuroprotective and disease-modifying properties. Researchers think that it may aid in the prevention of numerous neurodegenerative disorders, including Parkinson's disease, Alzheimer's disease, sleep disorders, and headaches.

  Studies have also proven that a diet high in fat and low in carbs even provide protection to the brain in strokes and traumatic brain injuries.

- *Lessen the Risk of Diabetes* – Ingesting carbs will cause a rapid rise in your blood sugar levels. This prompts the pancreas to yield insulin that the body will use to distribute glucose to the cells. The glucose will either be burned for fuel or stored in the cells.

Eating carbs (specifically the processed variety) in excessive amounts will trigger constant spikes in your insulin and blood sugar levels. This, in turn, can lead to a wide array of problems including obesity, type 2 diabetes, and insulin resistance.

When on a keto diet, you mainly eat fat that does not affect your blood sugar levels, and it likewise does not cause a spike in your insulin levels. You are, in effect, lowering your risk for ailments linked to high blood sugar. Many people are able to discontinue or at least minimize their dependence on diabetes medication after following a ketogenic diet.

- *Lower the Risk of Metabolic Syndrome* – According to the National Heart, Lung, & Blood Institute, metabolic syndrome is a group of risk factors that elevates your exposure to heart disease, as well as other health concerns like stroke and diabetes.

  You will likely be diagnosed with metabolic syndrome if you have at least three of the five risk factors for the condition. These are:

  - Elevated blood pressure
  - High blood sugar
  - Low HDL or good cholesterol levels
  - Abdominal obesity

- High levels of triglyceride, which is a type of fat

Now, if having high levels of triglyceride is a risk factor, shouldn't it follow that a diet high in fat would not be good for you? The question may have a sound basis. However, a low carb keto diet alters the way the body processes fats.

Studies have shown that the diet is actually able to lessen abdominal fat and triglycerides more than a low-fat diet does. It can also decrease blood sugar levels, lower LDL cholesterol, and raise HDL cholesterol levels. This means the ketogenic diet lowers your risk of acquiring metabolic syndrome that may lead to diabetes, stroke, heart disease, as well as many other obesity-related health problems.

- Improve Endurance and Athletic Performance – In 2004, Ben Greenfield was part of the University of Connecticut's FASTER study, the purpose of which was to determine how a low-carb, high-fat diet can impact athletic performance. Participants were called keto-adapted, fat-adapted athletes.

Greenfield is considered as among the 100 Most Influential People in Fitness and Health. He is an ironman triathlete, bio-hacker, brain performance trainer, and New York Times bestselling author of the book "Beyond Training: Mastering Endurance, Health & Life."

During the months leading up to the study, Greenfield adopted a ketogenic diet. He then underwent a grueling series of physical challenges at UConn's Human Performance Laboratory that included blood tests, stool tests, saliva swabs, and thigh muscle tissue extraction and analysis.

The FASTER study conclusion was in consonance with what each and every keto diet practitioner hopes to find out: that compared to well-trained high-endurance athletes on HC diet, adopting the keto diet on a long term basis results to amazingly high-fat oxidation rates, and the muscle glycogen utilization as well as the repletion patterns throughout and following a 3-hr. run are the same.

The bottom line is simply this. Fat oxidation or the process of breaking down fat lipids into smaller chunks occur to facilitate energy conversion. The UConn research arrived at the conclusion that using the keto diet on a long-term basis helps well-trained high-endurance athletes raise the number of fats that they can break down and burn.

Greenfield provided four main takeaways from his participation in the study:

- Eating a fat-loaded diet will not make you fat.
- Eating a fat-loaded diet will provide more fat to burn fat for energy both during exercise and at rest.

    - Eating a fat-loaded diet will allow you to function or exercise for a longer time while consuming a relatively less amount of calories.

    - Avoiding the intake of a high-carb diet will improve health, but it will not compromise performance.

- *Lower Risk of Cancer* – This may be a bit of bad news for processed meat-lovers the world over, but it is not completely surprising. Recently, the World Health Organization (WHO) has classified processed meats under Group 1 carcinogen. According to WHO, the category applies in case there is sufficient evidence to believe the food item is carcinogenic to humans. To put it simply, enough convincing evidence is present to the effect that it may cause cancer. Likewise, the WHO identified all forms of red meat under Group 2A, which means they are "probably" carcinogenic to humans.

  As far as red meat is concerned, the classification is only based on limited evidence culled from epidemiological studies that showed positive links between consumption of red meat and the development of colorectal cancer, and strong mechanistic evidence.

  Because a vegan diet in any form is, without a doubt, meat-free, the risk of getting cancer from red or processed meat is nil.

In a nutshell, the proven benefits of a meat-free diet like weight loss (particularly around the abdominal area) that include improved energy, blood sugar control, and better endurance and performance are enough reason for people around the world to incorporate a keto diet into their daily regimen.

The vegan keto diet is practically the same as the ketogenic diet – except for one major difference. It eliminates all types of animal products from the diet; thus, potentially merging all the great benefits of both the keto and vegan diets. In the process, the risk of gaining cancer from red and processed meats are taken out of the equation.

Having said that, there are minimal studies focused solely on a vegan keto diet. In addition, although there is overwhelming anecdotal evidence coming from people who have followed and benefited from the vegan keto diet, studies have to be done to determine the long term effects.

Food Items to Avoid

To gain the optimum benefit from the vegan keto diet, you must lower your carb consumption significantly, and replace it with vegan protein sources and healthy fats. Animal products like meat, eggs, dairy, poultry, and seafood should be excluded from your diet.

Food items you need to avoid completely include the following:

Meat and poultry	Pork, beef, chicken, and turkey
Dairy	Butter, milk, yogurt
Eggs	Egg whites and yolks
Seafood	Shrimp, fish, mussels, clams
Animal-based ingredients	Honey, whey protein, egg white protein

You should significantly reduce your consumption of the following:

Starches and grains	Rice, bread, cereal, pasta, baked goods, grains
Sugary beverages	Soda, sweet tea, smoothies, juices, chocolate milk, sports drinks
Sweeteners	White and brown sugar, maple syrup, agave

Starchy veggies	Sweet potatoes, potatoes, beets, peas, winter squash
Legumes and beans	Chickpeas, kidney beans, black beans
Fruits	Consumption of all fruits must be limited.
High carb alcoholic drinks	Beer, wine, sweetened cocktail
Low-fat diet food	This type of food tends to contain high amounts of added sugar
High carb condiments and sauces	Sweetened salad dressings, barbecue sauce, marinades
Highly processed food	Limit consumption of packaged food, while increasing intake of unprocessed, whole food.

When on a vegan keto diet, the limit of your carb intake will depend on our particular needs and health goals. However, in general, vegan protein sources, as well as high-fat vegan foods should make up a big chunk of your regular diet.

As a rule, you must significantly restrict your intake of animal food products, and high carb foods like sweetened beverages, grains, and starchy veggies.

Food Items to Eat

The vegan keto diet involves eating primarily healthy food items low in carbs and high in fat.

Following are the types of food you need to consume when on a vegan keto diet:

Coconut products	Coconut cream, full-fat coconut milk, unsweetened coconut
Oils	Nut oil, avocado oil, olive oil, MCT oil
Seeds and nuts	Brazil nuts, almonds, hemp seeds, walnuts, macadamia nuts, chia seeds, pumpkin seeds
Seed and nut butter	Almond butter, peanut butter, cashew butter, sunflower butter

Non-starchy veggies	Leafy greens, broccoli, Brussels sprouts, zucchini, peppers, mushrooms, cauliflower
Vegan sources of protein	Tempeh, full-fat tofu
Vegan full-fat dairy	Vegan butter, coconut yogurt, vegan cream cheese, cashew cheese
Avocados	Guacamole, whole avocados
Berries	Blueberries, raspberries, blackberries, strawberries (but only in moderation)
Condiments	Fresh herbs, nutritional yeast, salt & pepper, lemon juice, other spices

Although the ketogenic diet eliminates a lot of food groups that a vegan relies on, like starchy vegetables and whole grains, you can still adopt a vegan keto diet. You can do this with careful planning of your meals.

To replace the calories you will lose from avoiding highly processed and non-vegan foods, you can increase your consumption of unprocessed, whole foods.

Disadvantages and Side Effects of a Vegan Keto Diet

While a vegan keto diet may bring health benefits, it may also pose some potential downsides. For one, your diet will result in deficiencies in some important nutrients. This is particularly true if you fail to plan carefully.

A vegan keto diet often lacks in vitamins B12, D, and K2, as well as in omega 3 fats, zinc, calcium, and iron. It is crucial that you replace nutrient deficiencies with supplements and high-quality food.

Disadvantages

As it is, a vegan diet is already restrictive. You can expect a vegan keto diet to be even more restrictive. When you follow the diet, it is important that you supplement your meals with quality vitamins and minerals. This will help make sure that your meals are nutritionally adequate.

You need to eat fortified foods, focus on whole foods, and enhance nutrient availability through sprouting and fermenting. Nevertheless, it would be difficult to get all your micronutrient requirements from food alone.

As mentioned, supplementing with specific minerals and vitamins that are often missing in a vegan diet is a great way to avert potential nutrient deficiencies. This will also help you meet your daily nutritional needs.

Side Effects

By now, you should be aware that it would be difficult to transition into a keto diet. The time it takes to shift from a high-carb to a ketogenic diet can take a toll on your body. You may experience what is known as “keto flu.”

As your body goes through the transition from burning and using glucose for fuel to fat, your body will begin to experience unpleasant symptoms. These include nausea, fatigue, irritability, poor concentration, diarrhea, constipation, headaches, weakness, dizziness, muscle cramps, and difficulty in sleeping.

You can help ease these keto flu symptoms by keeping your body hydrated, consuming foods rich in fiber, engaging in light activities, and getting enough rest each day.

In addition, supplementing with electrolytes like magnesium, potassium, and sodium can help relieve specific symptoms like headaches, insomnia, and muscle pains.

Because the vegan keto diet has many food restrictions, it follows that it may not be the appropriate diet for everyone. It is not recommended for nursing or pregnant women, people with type 1 diabetes, athletes, and people with known eating disorders or a history thereof.

When considering shifting to a vegan keto diet, make sure to consult with your physician or a qualified health practitioner first. This way, you can sure, that the diet will be safe for you to follow.

Easy Ways to Add a Plant-Based Diet

Following are some tips on how to make the transition to a plant-based diet easy:

1. Don't give up everything in one go. – When adopting a new diet regimen, it is always best to start gradually, especially if the change is significant, such as eliminating all meat and dairy products in your regular fare.

   Start the diet shift slowly. For example, you can replace meat for 1 day in a week, and then increase the number of meatless days later. Do not hurry, as this will only make the risk of quitting the diet higher.

2. Watch out for refined carbs. – When giving up meat, especially during the initial stages, you may tend to replace protein deficiency with refined carbs. Sadly, they would not make up for the meat. Worse, they contain many calories.

To avoid overeating carbs, fill your pantry with healthy snacks like celery and baby carrots that you can serve with hummus or other tasty bean dips. Do not wait for hunger pangs to creep in, as you may be tempted to go for refined carbs.

3. Make a vegan version of your favorite dish. – Going from a meat-based to a plant-based diet can be difficult, especially if you think about no longer enjoying your favorite dishes. However, with a bit of research, you will be pleasantly surprised that most of your favorite meals, if not all, have a vegan version.

   You love tacos, for example, but it is not allowed on a vegan keto diet, you can prepare a meat-free version by substituting the meat with some Portobello mushrooms. Many vegan ingredients are among the best brain foods around. Thus, you will not only enjoy your favorite meal but many other health benefits as well.

4. Treat your cookbook as your best friend. – Especially, when starting your transition to a plant-based diet, you will need to rely a lot more on your cookbook.

   While you can find lots of recipes online, a cookbook is typically more organized. It can cover your needs more efficiently. In addition, a good cookbook can open the doors for you to learn various cooking styles. This way, you can add more variety to your meals.

5. Do some research by visiting some vegan restaurants! – Eating out will allow you to discover many vegan ingredients you did not know existed. So, if you think eating out is only an unnecessary luxury, better think again.

6. Veggies and fruits can be versatile. – At the start, you may find your plant-based diet boring, especially when you only know a few recipes. However, with a little imagination, you will find out that fruits and veggies can be quite versatile.

   Try to look at plants from a different perspective. For instance, instead of preparing zucchini the traditional way, turn it into pasta, then create a delicious meal from it. On the other hand, you can use them to make mouth-watering desserts, smoothies, or just add them to water for a healthy and refreshing drink.

7. Talk with a friend who has been on the same diet for a long time. – It is always a good idea to get advice from someone who has been there and done that. Who knows, they might be able to share their knowledge on recipes, meals, and ingredients you can add to your menu. They may also be able to teach you which restaurants to visit, and where to shop.

8. Variety is key. – Yes, you may have given up meat, but that does not mean your new diet is monotonous. You can enjoy a

wide variety of dishes that include fruits, vegetables, legumes, seeds, nuts, and a host of other plant-based ingredients.

Just make sure to read the labels for the nutritional content of your meals. This way, you can avoid consuming an excessive amount of calories in a single meal.

9. Prepare delicious vegan desserts. – Who says vegan desserts are boring and bland? Do your research, and look for plant-based ingredients that you can use to create mouth-watering desserts.

   For one, you can make delicious vegan mistakes using maple graham crust with silken tofu as filling. You can also create apple spice cake with added maple buttercream for a distinctive taste.

10. Find healthy meat alternatives to help you through tough days. – The internet provides access to information about a wide array of healthy meatless options. It would be a waste not to use it.

    Some of the best meat alternatives are seitan, tempeh, edamame beans, and tofu. Each one is a good source of healthy plant-based protein and is a good substitute for meat protein. In addition, the can offer new flavors for more exciting new options.

Try these tips to help make your transition to a vegan keto diet smooth and hassle-free. The key is to do some research on the processes, recipes, and ingredients you can use. Be bold, and try as many recipes as you can prepare, and have a lot of fun experimenting.

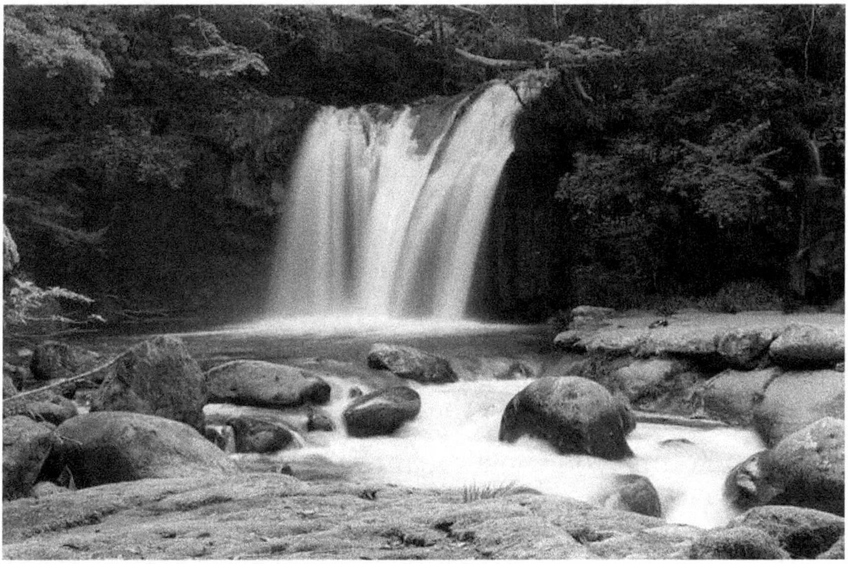

Preparing for the New Metabolism

The transition from glucose dependence for fuel to metabolism that relies primarily on fat-based fuel sources is known as keto-adaptation. During this phase, fat oxidation will not only increase. Your body will also begin to produce a significant amount of ketones to use as an additional source of fuel.

Ketones come from the fat that is partially metabolized. Like glucose, ketones can be used in different body tissues, including a significant part of the brain. Using ketones and fat offer a lot more benefits compared to using glucose. However, your metabolism will likely take time to adjust to generating and using ketones at a higher rate.

There will be visible changes within a few days after you begin restricting your carb intake. However, the improvements will continue for several weeks to come.

Following are some of the important facts about keto-adaptation that you can prepare for:

- Carb-based fueling is a cycle that self-perpetuates. It depletes fast, and each time you consume more carbs, you delay your adaptation to fat-based fueling.
- Fat burning, on the other hand, is sustainable. It provides access to a massive energy store without requiring you to stop often to refuel. Your blood sugar levels are maintained through efficient internal processes. Thus, you will not experience wild swings. All these results to a stable and even flow of energy, as well as improved mood and alertness.
- You will experience a delay or lull from the time you first reduce your carb intake and achieving a smooth-running fat

metabolism. In the day's in-between, you may feel sluggish, slow, or sometimes unwell.

To minimize the symptoms, make sure to keep hydrated, consume a lot of healthy fat, and liberally using salt. You can also find adding other electrolytes helpful. For one, a homemade broth is a great supplement.

Maintain low-carb consumption on a consistent basis. Otherwise, your body may take longer to adapt to the new metabolism – or it may not get there at all. The entire process will just go on and on for an indefinite period.

Be Careful Eating Out: Keto Vegan Diet Eating Out Tips

Following a vegan keto diet and giving up meat does not mean saying goodbye to dining out as well. Whether you are celebrating with family or friends, having dinner in a relative's home, or taking a quick lunch during a work break, you can maintain your diet and still enjoy low-carb meals through the following tips.

The basics of Eating Out

- Plan ahead. – A lot of restaurants today post their menu on their websites. If you are new to vegan keto, and you are worried about not finding anything suitable to eat, have a look at the online menu first before you go. Look for entries that are keto-friendly, which are likely to be delicious and sugar-free. Once you arrive at the restaurant, check if you can customize your order to make it ideal for you low-carb regiment.

- Get rid of the starch. – You can avoid the temptation of eating starchy food by keeping them off your plate. Order your meal, if possible, sans the starchy sides. Shun the pasta, bread, potatoes, and rice.

  Most restaurants would gladly replace the starch in an entrée with extra vegetables or a salad. When ordering a burger or sandwich, ask if you can substitute the bun with a lettuce wrap. If the restaurant does not allow substitution, then just remove the unwanted items from your plate once your order arrives.

  Even after ordering carefully, you may still get a plate with starchy sides. In that case, you have the option to just leave it untouched. However, if you feel that you will be tempted to have some of it, ask the waiter politely to re-plate the dish without the starch. In more casual dining places, you may need to remove the unnecessary items yourself.

- Include healthy fat. – Some restaurant dishes are low in fat, and you may find them less filling when eaten without carbs. You can address the problem by simply adding fat to the standard fare. You can ask for some extra butter for your veggies, or some vinegar dressing and olive oil for your salad.

There are restaurants that use cheaper vegetable oils, instead of olive oil. This is not good for your diet. To be on the safe side, always bring a small container of olive oil with you.

When ordering tea or coffee, ask for heavy cream to go with your beverage.

You should also watch out for condiments and sauces. Béarnaise sauce, for example, is mostly fat, while ketchup contains mostly carbs. To be sure, ask about the sauce ingredients. Shun it if it has flour, sugar, and other starchy thickeners. Request to have your sauce on the side. This way, you can control the amount to include in your meal.

- Choose your drinks carefully. - Safe choices include water, coffee, tea, and sparkling water. If you wish to have an alcoholic beverage, great low-carb options include dry wine, light beer, champagne, or spirits.
- Decide on whether or not to have dessert. – If you are no longer hungry, you may forego dessert, and just have a nice cup of tea or coffee as you wait for the others to finish off their desserts. If you think it is late to have coffee, ask for the decaf variety or some herbal tea instead.

Now, if you are still hungry, and still want to eat, ask for berries with heavy cream or a cheese plate. In most cases, however, adding butter or cream in your coffee would be sufficient.

- Use your creativity, if necessary. – If you find nothing suitable to order on the menu, you can try improvising. For example, you can order a couple of keto-friendly appetizers instead of an entrée. Pair a salad with shrimp cocktail, then add a cheese plate for a complete low-carb meal.

The key is to ask. As the customer, you deserve to get the meal you desire. However, always ask in a nice, polite way.

Getting Your Family Involved with Plant-Based Diet

Like all other long-term sustainable changes, the process of getting your entire family involved with a plant-based diet must be done at a slow and steady pace – with a lot of creativity. After all, convincing an entire household on the benefits of plant-based diets is a lot tougher than a single person adopting the change.

The first step would be to educate your family on the reasons you want to make the transition. Present it in a way that they will appreciate all the benefits they stand to enjoy. This way, they will be willing to try it, at the very least.

Once you have convinced everybody that the diet would be good for everyone, make sure to implement the change gradually. For instance, you can start by preparing plant-based meals for one day a week. Then, increase the number of plant-based days in the following weeks until the entire family gets comfortable with vegan meals for the entire week.

Making a complete shift within a short period may be too overwhelming for your family, and may cause them to become divided about the diet.

In the meantime, you can start looking for various recipes that you can use. This can be particularly useful, especially if you do not have much experience in preparing plant-based meals. This will also ensure variety as you slowly introduce the diet to your household. After all, you would not want your loved ones to think that the new regimen means having to eat boiled cauliflower and broccoli day in and day out.

By having a wide range of recipes in your arsenal, you will also eliminate one of the biggest barriers to a smooth transition. As you learn how to effectively use different plants in all your dishes, you will realize that plant-based dishes can be as delectable and satisfying as their meat-based counterparts.

You will discover that simple cooking techniques like sautéing or oven-roasting vegetables can go a long way in providing texture and flavor to your meals.

While it may take some time before you master and perfect preparing plant-based meals, it will be worth all the effort. In the meantime, just enjoy exploring and experimenting in the kitchen.

In time, you will learn how to prepare textured and flavorful plant-based dishes that your entire family will begin to love.

Finding Your Carbohydrate Tolerance Level

There is a good reason why the keto diet is taking the world by storm. After all, the low-carb, high-fat philosophy that the diet adheres to is known for its weight loss and anti-inflammatory benefits, as well as its overall contribution to better health and wellbeing.

While these benefits may seem on the "magical" side, there actually is no magic involved. They are simply the result of how keto makes your body shift from getting its energy from glucose (the traditional energy source) to ketones. Because the diet is low in carb, glucose will not be available. Thus, the liver will instead produce ketones.

The idea is quite simple. Get the body into a state of ketosis. The problem is, getting into that state can be a complex process. To make the body use ketones and not glucose, you need to limit your carb intake – drastically. Your body will then need to undergo a transition period to learn how to get energy from an alternative source.

Getting into ketosis takes anywhere between two days and two weeks, depending on the diet you were eating before adopting the keto diet, as well as other personal circumstances. It is worth mentioning that it is not like other elimination diets that once you commit to it, you can no longer quit – without repercussions.

When in ketosis, you become metabolically flexible. This means your cells can use various sources of energy. They can use glucose, and they can use fats and switch getting energy between the two. There would be no problem either way.

It is also not necessary for you to get to ketosis each day of your life. That is not the goal. You can get in and out anytime.

The key is to have the right balance between adding fat in your diet that is enough for the body to generate ketones and limiting your carb intake to an amount that is enough for your body to consume ketones for energy, instead of glucose.

The number of carbs you need to limit your intake to depends on three primary factors:

1. *The type of carbs you include on your keto diet* – While you significantly lower your carb intake because of the keto diet, you cannot eliminate it. After all, there are carbs in almost any food you eat – from fruits to grains to veggies. Even protein will eventually convert into glucose. This means the keto diet likewise limits protein.

   A healthy ketogenic diet is not just about eating fat generously. It is about combining liberal amounts of healthy fats with nutrient-rich low-carb whole foods. This means consuming lots of veggies as well.

   Like sugar and grains, vegetables also contain carbohydrate. However, they also contain essential vitamins, phytonutrients, and minerals. To be specific, consuming veggies rich in fiber such as sweet peas, artichokes, okra, and parsnips in moderation can be quite helpful. These veggies do not trigger blood sugar level spikes unlike simple carbs like sugar.

   It is likewise important to monitor your intake of certain minerals like magnesium, potassium, and sodium. This is because when your body switches energy sources from carbs to fat, your kidneys likewise shift from retaining to excreting sodium together with other minerals like magnesium.

   Experts say that consuming 3 to 7 g of sodium each day is all right. Healthy sources are from pink Himalayan or sea salt.

Almonds, pumpkin, and spinach are good sources of magnesium, while you can get your potassium from avocados.

Supplementing is also recommended. Taking multivitamins daily, as well as 300 – 500 mg of magnesium glycinate or magnesium citrate, and about 1300 – 3500 mg potassium citrate can be helpful.

Another important step is to always stay hydrated. Dehydration is a possible side effect of the ketogenic diet. Drinking at least 2.5 liters of water each day will help relieve the effects of the diet's early stages. These include constipation and headaches.

When on keto, fermented foods are also important to ensure good digestive health. It is therefore good to add sauerkraut or kimchi, as well as probiotics to your diet.

2. *Net carbs vs. total carbs* – Most keto experts recommend a carb intake of about 20 g of net carbs when on the diet. Net carbs are the number of carbs in grams of a particular food item less the fiber in grams. To achieve that level, you can use a calorie counter app to compute for the exact amount of net carbs you are consuming on a daily basis.

   You can start with what is known as the "Feast Phase" where you include a lot more fat without restricting protein or carbs for three days. Then, you adjust your macros to suit a fully keto diet. This means getting around 60 – 75% of your calorie consumption from high-quality fats. You get 20 – 30% from protein sources, and the remaining 5 – 10% from carbs.

The exact amount of net carbs will vary between individuals, but most will fall within the range of 20 – 50 net carbs a day. Typically, it is ideal for women to stay within the range of 20 -30 g each day, and 30 – 50 g for men, unless you are trying to cut calories dramatically.

It is not recommended to cut back on carb consumption in one go. Starting with 100 g would be a good idea, and then gradually reducing your consumption until you get to your target level.

Making sustainable and small shifts to lower carb consumption is longer lasting and more effective compared to jumping right away to 20 carbs each day from a standard regular diet of around 100+ carbs a day.

A sudden drastic change can also result in "keto flu," making you feel lethargic and tired as your body frantically searches for energy. This typically happens when the body is in a transition phase from a carbohydrate-based metabolism to one based on facts.

3. *Counting or improvising* – Bear in mind that strict carb targets are mere jump-off points. Each one has their own

carb tolerance for keto that they need to determine on their own. Many experts recommend beginning by religiously counting the grams of carbs.

Another recommendation is to strictly stick to an extremely low number for around 60 days, then start to gradually consume more carbs as the body learns to use ketones more efficiently. How many carbs would that depend on various factors like fitness level, lean muscle mass, and insulin tolerance! Everyone is different and thus needs to find their own sweet spot.

There are two popular methods of finding your carb tolerance. First is using the ketone monitor. It measures ketone levels in the urine, blood, or breath. Although this can provide good results, many experts instead recommend learning how to listen properly to your body. Since carb tolerance is personal in nature, the best indicator is how you are feeling, ruling out trial and error, and medical conditions.

To determine where you stand after you have reduced your intake to the minimum, experiment with moderately carb-rich food such as ½ sweet potato to go with a keto-friendly dinner. Wait a few hours, then test your ketones using a ketone monitor, or observe how you are feeling to check if you are still in ketosis.

By experimenting with various foods in this manner, you will soon learn to manage your keto diet without having to rely on your calorie counting app and ketone monitor. This way, the diet will be more sustainable for you.

A low-carb diet is a lifestyle. It is a healthy, balanced, and good way to eat. So keep it simple.

Determining Your Personal Protein Threshold

Whether you are adopting the keto diet for health or to lose weight, finding the appropriate protein level can be quite confusing, especially for a beginner. To achieve a relatively smooth keto-adaptation, experts recommend a caloric spread of 70 to 80% fat, 15 to 25% protein, and 5% carbs from fibrous, green veggies. However, this may vary, depending on individual circumstances. Thus, it can be misleading and confusing.

The best way to check micronutrients is in grams – and not in percentages. After all, there is no one magic number or ratio. Your personal protein threshold depends on your particular preferences, needs, and goals. These will determine how much protein you will need for your keto diet. It often falls somewhere between 1 to 2.2 kg of body weight or even higher in some cases, or ½ to 1 lb. of lean body mass.

Variables That Have an Effect on Your Optimal Protein Intake

Keto for Weight Loss

1. *You are Personal Goals* – Protein plays a vital role in macronutrient partitioning. It is the process of breaking down calories from protein, carbs, and fat as a percentage of your total daily calorie consumption.

   If your target is to lose fat, you need to maintain a calorie deficit so your body can tap into your fat reserves for energy. One way to make the deficit sustainable, and to some extent, even fun, is through a keto diet. When properly formulated, the diet will have sufficient amounts of protein and fiber-rich veggies to fill your tummy, and curb hunger, while keeping your blood sugar levels more stable compared to a carb-based diet.

   When you are in a calorie deficit, protein can be a potent tool to increase satiety. You can make the deficit more bearable by increasing your protein intake while dropping fat consumption. This will create the necessary energy balance that can trigger a necessity to burn fat reserves the whole day through. Increased protein levels can also help normalize levels of insulin in calorie-restricted diets for obese hyperinsulinemic people.

   For weight loss goals, ideal protein levels may range from 1.5 to 2.5 g per kg of lean body mass. The recommended range is wide. Thus, you need to do some experimentation in order to determine your optimal intake.

If you are physically active you will likely require more protein than if you lead a sedentary lifestyle. In general, men often want more protein than women do. However, there is no compelling reason to consume 1.5 g per kg of lean body mass just to get lean if you are following a keto regimen.

The low end of the keto spectrum may not bring the desired muscle loss since ketosis spares the muscles, and protects lean muscles from catabolism. However, it is not crucial to severely limit the protein consumption of people under a medical keto diet such as epileptic patients. If you love to eat protein, and highly active, the high end of the keto spectrum is not recommended protein. If you want to eat less protein, then, by all means, limit your protein intake.

Keto Diet for Medical Reasons

If you want to maintain a medical keto regimen, and higher levels of blood ketones at all times, while minimizing MTOR and IGF-1 as much as you can, then you will most likely favor intake levels in the lower end of the keto spectrum.

Keeping low levels of mTOR and IGF-1 while increasing AMPK is an important health strategy that you can use even if you are not suffering from any serious ailment. Deep ketosis is quite helpful for epileptics because of its neuroprotective properties that affect the brain.

Recent findings are beginning to show how the diet can be an effective metabolic for cancer as well. If ketosis is a necessary metabolic therapy for serious health conditions, it is crucial to maintain low protein levels to raise blood ketone, and keep levels of blood sugar very low. For serious ailments, low consumption of protein, such as 1 g per kg of lean body mass, may not be needed.

This does not mean people on a higher protein diet will not gain any of the known benefits of ketosis. However, when intended to be a metabolic therapy for patients of serious diseases, the diet can be difficult to maintain because it is more restrictive than a keto diet intended for the average person. Note that this book is not meant to be a medical keto diet resource. As such, if you are using keto for medical purposes, it is best to consult with your physician first.

2. *Dietary History* – When choosing your appropriate protein intake, it is important to consider your dietary history. Especially if you have never had sufficient protein in your diet. It would be difficult for you to adjust to an intake level at the high end of the keto spectrum.

If you have adapted to keto well, and you experience stable levels of energy the entire day without experiencing hunger a lot, you can increase your protein intake a little, and lower your fat consumption. This will help create more satiety, as well as a bit deeper calorie deficit that can help facilitate improved fat burning.

If you have never been under a diet before, and you have a condition known as blood sugar dysregulation, you may benefit from starting with either a higher or lower protein intake, depending on other health history and lifestyle factors. Again, there is no one-size-fits-all "magic amount" of protein consumption to achieve.

3. *Level of Activity* – A more active person will more likely have a lot faster metabolism compared to a less active individual. Thus, they may experience feeling hungry more often. If you are on the active side, you will tend to desire a higher protein intake than if you are sedentary. Being less active, you will have less requirement for gluconeogenesis substrate since your metabolism will be slower, utilizing less glucose for physical activities and explosive movements.

   You may find this surprising, but resistance training is actually muscle sparing, meaning it reduces your protein requirements. However, the more you restrict your calories, the bigger the amount of protein you will need to spare your lean tissues. Therefore, if you are an active individual, and you want to get lean, consuming is both desired as well as required, in particular, if you are under a significant calorie deficit.

The state of ketosis is muscle sparing. However, you need to produce glucose for your brain and muscle glycogen. Thus, more training means more protein. Evidence is mounting to the effect that a higher protein intake while on a diet can improve the outcome. As always, it is safer to be at the higher end of the spectrum.

Sedentary people may want only 1 to 1.5 g per kg of lean body mass. More active people, on the other hand, may go for 1.5 to 2.5 g per kg of lean body mass.

4. Personal Preferences - many people – even health coaches – often forget this factor. Ironically, this is among the most important of the lot. If you love eating protein, but you have no access to enough fresh salmon, for example, then maybe it is a good idea to turn your attention to the high end of the keto spectrum for protein.

   Your own personal preference is a major factor if you intend to stick to the diet for the long term. This means you need to enjoy the diet you put your commitment to in order to get the results you want. If you want lots of protein, you can follow the higher end of the spectrum. Eat 1.6 to 2.2 g of protein for every kg. Of your LBM.

You can go a bit higher if you are very active and you really want more protein. You have to realize, however, that you may reach the limit where you will start oxidizing protein as a source of energy, and it may upregulate the pathways.

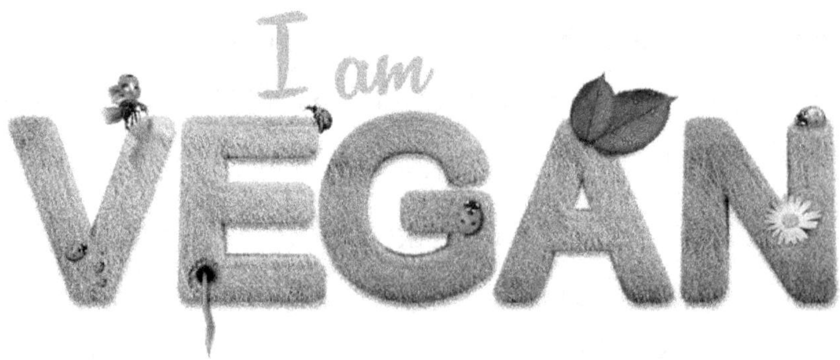

Chapter 3: The Vegan Keto Shopping List and Sample Meal Plan

The Vegan Keto Shopping List

Regardless of whether you have been on the vegan keto diet for only a few weeks, or you have religiously been following the regimen for over a year now, there is always a new ingredient that is just waiting for you to discover! While shopping for your keto ingredients, how many times did you say to yourself "I never realized this item is low carb?"

The following list contains a comprehensive breakdown of all available vegan keto food items out there for you to explore and enjoy. You do not necessarily have to buy everything on the list to survive on a low-carb, whole-food, plant-based diet. We feel you need to know everything, and have it available, just in case. Some of the items may not be available in some areas, or during certain seasons.

Here are some notes to keep in mind before you check out the list:

- Items with an asterisk (*) marking have a bit high carb content, and you should consume them sparingly.
- Items with a (P) marking are great protein sources.
- All items are often available in most American and Canadian supermarkets.

Vegan Keto Fats	Nuts	Almonds (P)
		Cashews*
		Brazil nuts

		Macadamia nuts
		Hazelnuts/filberts
		Peanuts
		Pecans
		Pistachios*
		Pine nuts*
		Walnuts
	Seeds	Hemp seeds (P)
		Sunflower seeds
		Chia seeds
		Pumpkin seeds
	Nut and Seed Butters	Coconut butter/coconut manna
		Almond butter (P)
		Macadamia nut butter
		Peanut butter (P)
		Hazelnut butter

		Tahini
		Sunflower seed butter
	Other Whole Food Sources of Fat	Coconut
		Olives
		Avocados
	Healthy Oils	Avocado oil
		Coconut oil
		Cacao butter (well-suited for desserts and body care
		Almond oil
		Flaxseed oil (not for cooking; best stored cold)
		Macadamia nut oil
		Hazelnut oil
		Walnut oil

		MCT oil
		Olive oil
Low Carb Fruits and Veggies	Low carb veggies	Arugula
		Asparagus
		Artichoke hearts
		Beets*
		Bell peppers (green variety is lowest in carb content)
		Brussels sprouts*
		Broccoli
		Bok choy
		Carrots*
		Cauliflower
		Cabbage
		Celeriac/celery root
		Celery

		Collards
		Chard
		Daikon radish
		Cucumbers
		Eggplant
		Dandelion greens
		Endive/escarole
		Fiddleheads (available only in spring, and for brief periods)
		Fennel
		Jicama*
		Kale*
		Lettuce (all kinds)
		Mushrooms
		Onion*
		Okra

		Mustard greens
		Rhubarb
		Radish
		Spinach
		Shallots
		Swiss chard
		Summer type squash
		Winter type squash (pumpkin, butternut, spaghetti)
		Zucchini
		Turnips
	Low Carb Fruits	Blueberries*
		Avocado
		Lemon
		Coconut
		Cranberries

		Lime
		Lemon
		Strawberries
		Raspberries
		Olives
		Watermelon*
		Tomatoes
Pantry Supplies		Baking powder
		Almond flour
		Baking soda
		Baking powder
		Cocoa or cacao powder
		Coconut flour
		Coconut milk
		Dark chocolate (85% or more is often low in sugar

		Hearts of palm
		Glucomannan powder
		Psyllium husk
		Jackfruit (in brine, and not syrup)
		Vanilla extract (no sugar)
		Nutritional yeast
Vegan Fridge Staples		Dairy-free yogurt* (unsweetened, any type)
		Apple cider vinegar
		Dairy-free cheese
		Micro-greens
		Pickles (sugar-free)
		Seitan (P)
		Sprouts (all kinds)
		Sauerkraut/vegan

		kimchi
		Tofu (P)
		Tempeh (P)
Other Vegan Keto Staples		Various herbs & spices
		Kelp flakes
		Kelp noodles
		Edamame
		Lupine beans/lupins
		Nori sheets
		Shirataki noodles
		Roasted seaweed snacks
Sauces & Condiments		Mustard
		hot sauce/chili sauce
		Coconut aminos/ soy sauce tamari

		Tomato sauce
		Wasabi paste
		Vinegar (white wine, rice wine, balsamic)
Smoothie Add-Ins		Beetroot powder*
		Moringa
		Chlorella
		Turmeric
		Spirulina
Useful Gadgets to Have		High-quality food processor
		Grinder/Nutribullet
		Spiralizer
		Tofu press

You will find this list quite useful. Have it printed out, and keep a copy in your shopping bag. This way, you will always have a handy reference whenever you need to replenish your pantry for vegan keto-friendly supplies and ingredients and help you avoid buying things you do not really need.

One Week Vegan Ketogenic Diet Meal Plan

As you know, vegan keto may be a very restrictive diet. However, it does not mean you will easily run out of meals to prepare while following the diet. You can, in fact, prepare a wide variety of delicious meals using vegan-friendly ingredients.

Here is a sample one-week plan for the vegan ketogenic diet:

Sunday	Breakfast	Ketogenic Crispy Flaxseed Waffles
	Lunch	Low-Carb Noodle Bowls w/ Creamy Curry Sauce
	Dinner	Vegan Keto Carbonara
Monday	Breakfast	Green Coffee Shake
	Lunch	Vegan Caesar Salad Quick and Easy
	Dinner	Vegan Mushroom

		Burgers
Tuesday	Breakfast	Keto Overnight Oats
	Lunch	Asian-Style Spiralized Zucchini Salad
	Dinner	Mustard Dill Zucchini Cakes
Wednesday	Breakfast	Keto Pumpkin Latte Overnight Oats
	Lunch	Creamy Roasted Red Pepper Soup
	Dinner	Vegan Keto Sushi Bowl
Thursday	Breakfast	Grain-Free Keto Hemp Heart Porridge
	Lunch	Kelp Noodles w/ Avocado Pesto
	Dinner	Vegan Keto Bibimbap

Friday	Breakfast	Rocket Fuel Keto Iced Blended Coffee
	Lunch	One-Pot Zucchini Pasta
	Dinner	Cauliflower Pizza Crust, Low-Carb Vegan-Style
Saturday	Breakfast	Nut-Free, Grain-Free Keto Hemp Heart Porridge
	Lunch	Harissa Portobello Mushroom Tacos
	Dinner	Sloppy Joes, Vegan Keto Version

Vegan Keto Snacks

For snacks or if you feel hungry in-between meals, you can try any of the following healthy vegan keto fares:

- Nuts and coconut bars

- Sliced cucumbers topped w/ vegan cream cheese
- Coconut fat bombs (made w/ coconut oil, coconut butter, and shredded coconut)
- Cocoa and coconut milk smoothie
- Dried coconut flakes
- Trail mix 2/ mixed seeds, nuts, and unsweetened coconut
- Almond butter-topped celery sticks
- Coconut cream w/ berries
- Roasted pumpkin seeds
- Chopped almonds-topped coconut milk yogurt
- Cauliflower tater tots
- Guacamole w/ sliced bell peppers
- Olives stuffed w/ vegan cheese

Chapter 4: Vegan Keto Breakfast Recipes

Ketogenic Crispy Flaxseed Waffles

Serves: 4 Total Time: 25 min

Ingredients:

- 2 cups of golden flaxseed, roughly ground
- 5 Tbsp. of flaxseed finely ground + 15 Tbsp. of warm water
- 1 tsp. of sea salt
- ½ cup of water
- 1 cup of avocado
- 2 tsp. of ground cinnamon

Instructions:

1. Mix 5 Tbsp. of finely ground flaxseed and 15 Tbsp. of warm water. Allow sitting for about 5 minutes or until gooey.
2. Set the waffle maker to medium heat, or your preferred setting to make crisp waffles.
3. Mix the roughly ground flaxseed with sea salt and baking powder in a large-sized bowl. Combine well by whisking, then set aside.

4. Put the flaxseed and water mixture you prepared in step 1 in a high-powered blender. Blend at high setting for about 30 seconds or until foamy. Transfer contents to the large bowl with the other ingredients.
5. Stir using a spatula until everything is well mixed. You should get a very fluffy consistency. Allow the mixture to sit for around 3 minutes.
6. Stir the ground cinnamon in.
7. Scoop the batter and transfer to the preheated waffle maker (you should be able to make four scoops, cooking one scoop at a time). Close the waffle maker lid. Allow to cook until done or when you hear the beep.
8. Repeat step 7 with the remaining batter.
9. Serve immediately.
10. If preferred, transfer the waffles to an airtight container, and then freeze. When frozen, the waffles can last for a few weeks. Just take out the waffles, then toast for a quick on the go breakfast.

Rocket Fuel Keto Iced Blended Coffee

Serves: 1 Total Time: 15 min

Ingredients:

- 1 ¾ cup of brewed coffee (regular or decaf, or your preferred tea)
- 10 g. of cacao butter (around 4 to 5 wafers
- 1 Tbsp. of almond butter or 2 tsp. of hemp hearts
- 1 Tbsp. of coconut or MCT oil
- 4 drops of stevia (alcohol-free)
- ¼ tsp. of ground cinnamon (if preferred)
- ¼ tsp. of ground vanilla bean (if preferred)
- 1 tsp. of cacao nibs
- 4 to 6 pcs. of ice cubes

Instructions:

1. Blend coffee, cacao butter, almond butter, stevia. Cinnamon, vanilla, and MCT oil together in a high-powered blender. Move contents to a jar, then refrigerate to completely cool. You can do it in the evening to have a chilled jar by morning.

2. Take the chilled jar out of the refrigerator, and then put contents back into the blender. Add 4 to 6 cubes of ice. Make sure to break the ice cubes up before adding to the coffee, in case you are not using a high-powered blender. This will keep your drink from heating up.
3. Blend until the ice cubes are crushed.
4. Pour contents into a jar. Top with cacao nibs and coconut whipped cream.
5. Serve and enjoy!

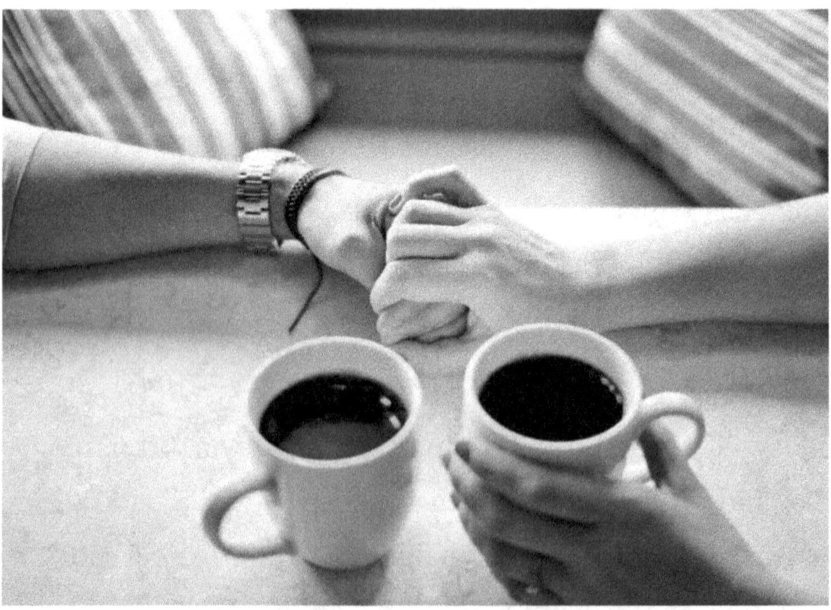

Green Coffee Shake

Serves: 4 Total Time: 5 min

Ingredients:

- 1 can (400 ml) of coconut milk (full-fat)
- 2 Tbsp. of almond butter (unsweetened)
- 1 ½ cup of chilled brewed coffee (regular or decaf)
- 1 Tbsp. of vanilla-flavored Genuine Health vegan greens
- 8 cubes of ice

Instructions:

1. Put all ingredients, except for the ice, in a blender. Process for about 10 seconds or until you achieve a smooth consistency.
2. Divide into 4 glasses, dropping 2 cubes of ice in each glass.
3. Serve and enjoy.

** Notes: In case there are leftovers, pour into airtight containers and refrigerate. It can last for 2 days. Just make sure to shake well before consuming

Chocolate Cinnamon Breakfast Smoothie

Serves: 1 Total Time: 5 min

Ingredients:

- ½ pc. of ripe avocado
- ¾ cup of coconut milk
- 1 tsp. of cinnamon powder
- 2 tsp. of cacao powder (unsweetened)
- ¼ tsp. of vanilla extract
- ½ tsp. of MCT oil or 1 tsp. of coconut oil, if preferred
- Stevia, if preferred

Instructions:

1. Put all ingredients in a blender and process well.
2. Transfer the contents in a tall glass.
3. Serve and enjoy!

Keto Overnight Oats

Serves: 2   Total Time: 5 min

Ingredients:

- 1 cup of coconut milk, full-fat (reserve ¼ cup to add the next day)
- 3 Tbsp. of hemp hearts
- 3 drops of liquid stevia (add more if preferred)
- 1 Tbsp. of chia seed
- 1 pinch of Himalayan rock salt, finely ground
- ½ tsp. of vanilla extract.

  For toppings (optional)

- 6 pcs. of whole raspberries
- 12 pcs. of whole almonds

Instructions:

1. Place all ingredients in at least a 350 ml container w/ a lid. Combine well by stirring. Cover the container, then refrigerate for at least 7 hours or leave overnight.
2. Take the container out of the refrigerator the next day. Add the reserved milk to achieve a nice consistency.
3. Transfer contents into two small-sized bowls. Add desired toppings.
4. Serve and enjoy!
5. Refrigerate any leftovers in an airtight container for up to two days.

Keto Fudge Overnight Oats

Serves: 2 Total Time: 5 min

Ingredients:

- 1 cup of coconut milk, full-fat (reserve ¼ cup to add the next day)
- 3 Tbsp. of hemp hearts
- 2 Tbsp. of cacao powder
- 1 Tbsp. of sunflower butter

- 3 drops of liquid stevia (add more if preferred)
- 1 Tbsp. of chia seed
- 1 pinch of Himalayan rock salt, finely ground
- ½ tsp. of vanilla extract.

For toppings (optional)

- Cacao nibs
- Unsweetened coconut, shredded
- Strawberries

Instructions:

1. Place all ingredients in at least a 350 ml container w/ a lid. Combine well by stirring. Cover the container, then refrigerate for at least 7 hours or leave overnight.
2. Take the container out of the refrigerator the next day. Add the reserved milk to achieve a nice consistency.
3. Transfer contents into two small-sized bowls. Add desired toppings.
4. Serve and enjoy!
5. Refrigerate any leftovers in an airtight container for up to two days.

Keto Pumpkin Latte Overnight Oats

Serves: 2 Total Time: 5 min

Ingredients:

- 3/4 cup of coconut milk, full-fat
- ¼ cup of brewed coffee (regular or decaf)
- 3 Tbsp. of hemp hearts
- 2 Tbsp. of canned pumpkin puree
- ¼ tsp. of pumpkin pie spice
- 3 drops of liquid stevia (add more if preferred)
- 1 Tbsp. of chia seed
- 1 pinch of Himalayan rock salt, finely ground
- ½ tsp. of vanilla extract.

  For toppings (optional)

- pecans
- additional ground cinnamon

Instructions:

1. Place all ingredients in at least a 350 ml container w/ a lid. Combine well by stirring. Cover the container, then refrigerate for at least 7 hours or leave overnight.
2. Take the container out of the refrigerator the next day. Add the reserved milk to achieve a nice consistency.
3. Transfer contents into two small-sized bowls. Add desired toppings.
4. Serve and enjoy!
5. Refrigerate any leftovers in an airtight container for up to two days.

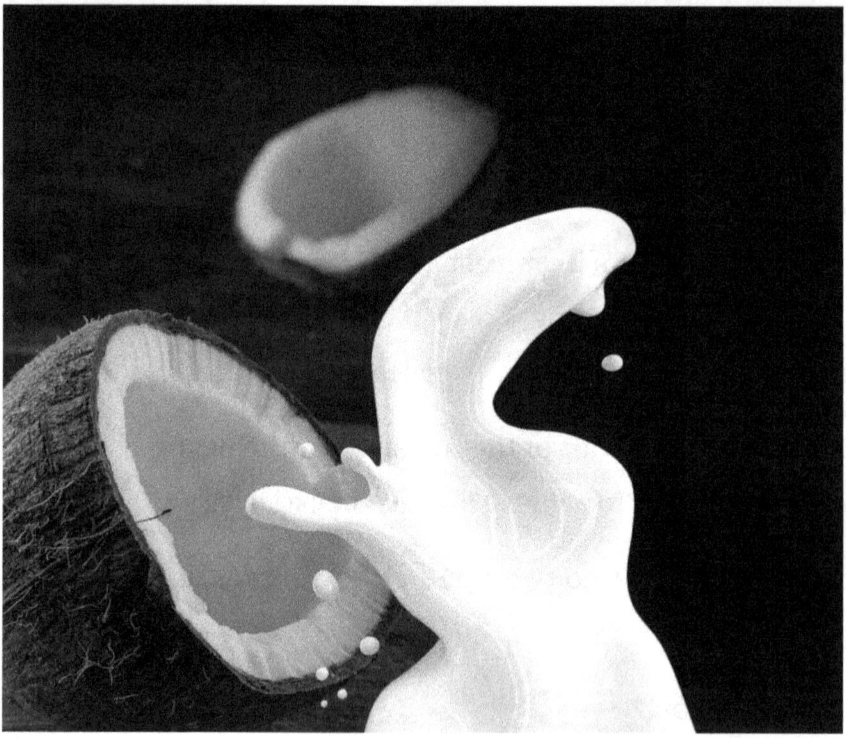

Vegan Keto Bagels

Serves: 6 (1 bagel per serving) Total Time: 50 min

Ingredients:

- ½ cup of tahini
- ½ cup of flaxseed, ground

- ¼ cup of psyllium husks
- 1 tsp. of baking powder
- 1 cup of water
- 1 pinch of salt (make it 1 tsp. if you are using unsalted tahini)
- Sesame seeds, for garnish.

Instructions:

1. Preheat the oven to 375° F.
2. Put flax seeds, baking powder, psyllium husks, and salt in a medium-sized mixing bowl. Combine the dry ingredients well by whisking thoroughly.
3. Get a separate bowl, and pour water into the tahini. Whisk thoroughly until the well combined.
4. Combine the dry ingredients with the wet ingredients. Stir well, and then form the dough by kneading. Knead everything thoroughly to make sure that the dough gets a uniform consistency.
5. Use your hand to form patties about 1/4" thick and 4" in diameter each. Lay down the patties on a baking tray. Make a small circle in the middle of each patty. You can use the larger end of a pastry tip (typically used for piping frosting) for the circles. Instead of a baking tray, you may prefer to use

a doughnut pan, if you think it would make the process easier.

6. Garnish with sesame seeds.
7. Put the tray in the oven, and allow baking for about 40 minutes, or until golden brown.
8. Cut the bread pieces into halves as you would a regular bagel.
9. Top with preferred toppings, and then serve.

Grain-Free Keto Hemp Heart Porridge

Serves: 1 Total Time: 5 min

Ingredients:

- 1 cup of non-dairy milk
- 2 Tbsp. of flaxseed, freshly ground
- ½ cup of hemp hearts
- 1 Tbsp. of chia seeds
- 5 drops of liquid stevia or 1 Tbsp. of xylitol
- ½ tsp. of ground cinnamon
- ¾ tsp. of pure vanilla extract.

- ¼ cup of crushed almonds (you can use almond flour if preferred)

For Toppings

- 3 pcs. of Brazil nuts
- 1 Tbsp. of hemp hearts

Instructions:

1. Place all the ingredients, except for the toppings and ground almonds in a small-sized saucepan. Stir thoroughly until everything is well combined. Heat the pan over medium heat setting or just as it starts to lightly boil. Leave the pan uncovered.
2. Once you see light bubbling, stir a little. Allow cooking for 1 to 2 minutes more.
3. Take the pan off the heat. Add the crushed almonds, and then stir.
4. Transfer the pan contents into a bowl. Put your desired toppings, and then serve right away.

Nut-Free, Grain-Free Keto Hemp Heart Porridge

Serves: 1   Total Time: 5 min

Ingredients:

- 1 cup of non-dairy milk
- 2 Tbsp. of flaxseed, freshly ground
- ½ cup of hemp hearts
- 1 Tbsp. of chia seeds
- 5 drops of liquid stevia or 1 Tbsp. of xylitol
- ½ tsp. of ground cinnamon
- ¾ tsp. of pure vanilla extract.
- ¼ cup of crushed sunflower seeds (you can use pumpkin seeds if preferred)

  For Toppings

- 3 pcs. of Brazil nuts
- 1 Tbsp. of hemp hearts

Instructions:

5. Place all the ingredients, except for the toppings and sunflower seeds in a small-sized saucepan. Stir thoroughly until everything is well combined. Heat the pan over medium heat setting or just as it starts to lightly boil. Leave the pan uncovered.
6. Once you see light bubbling, stir a little. Allow cooking for 1 to 2 minutes more.
7. Take the pan off the heat. Add the crushed almonds, and then stir.
8. Transfer the pan contents into a bowl. Put your desired toppings, and then serve right away.

Strawberry Chia Matcha Pudding

Serves: 1   Total Time: 5 min

Ingredients:

- 1 tsp. of matcha powder
- 1 ½ Tbsp. of chia seeds
- ¾ cup of coconut milk
- 2 pcs. of strawberries, diced into small pieces
- Raw honey or stevia, to taste (if preferred)

Instructions:

1. Put the matcha powder, chia seeds, and coconut milk together in a lidded cup. Add honey or stevia (if you prefer to use sweeteners). Shake thoroughly for about 5 to 10 seconds.
2. Pour the mixture into a tall glass. Refrigerate for about 4 hours.
3. Take the glass out of the refrigerator, and then stir in the diced strawberries. Set aside 1 tsp. of the diced strawberries for toppings.
4. When ready to serve, top with the reserved strawberries.
5. Enjoy!

Curried Tofu Scramble

Serves: 4 Total Time: 30 min

Equipment:

- Tofu press
- Large-sized sauté pan

Ingredients:

- 3 Tbsp. of low-sodium veggie broth (or water or olive oil, if preferred)
- 1 pc. of large-sized red pepper, diced
- ½ pc. of a medium-sized onion, diced
- 1 block of extra firm/firm organic tofu, pressed & drained
- 6 oz. of mushrooms, sliced
- 3 cups of greens (spinach, arugula, kale, dandelion greens), chopped
- Curry seasoning mix
- ½ tsp. of garlic powder
- ¼ tsp. of coriander
- ½ tsp. of cumin
- ½ tsp. of curry powder
- ¼ tsp. of turmeric (for color)
- ¼ tsp. of paprika
- ¼ tsp. of garam masala
- ¼ tsp. of black salt (or you can use Himalayan pink sea salt if preferred)

- 1 Tbsp. of water (for mixing the seasonings together to make a sauce)

Instructions:

1. Sauté onions in veggie broth in a large-sized pan for about 5 minutes. Add the mushrooms and red peppers, and cook for around 10 minutes.
2. Push aside the vegetables to one side of the pan. Place the pressed & drained tofu block on the pan is other side. Use a spatula to break it up into smaller chunks. Sauté for about 3 minutes.
3. Combine all seasonings in a small-sized bowl. Add just enough amount of water to allow you to whisk everything together. Pour the mix over the tofu pieces. Toss until all the pieces are coated. Combine the veggies and tofu, and mix well.
4. Add the greens. Put the pan cover on, and allow cooking for about 5 mins. Alternatively, until the greens start to wilt.
5. Top with hot sauce and green onions.
6. Serve hot and enjoy right away!

**Notes: It is important to press the tofu, and drain the water out. Otherwise, you will be left with a spongy tofu scramble.

Using a tofu press is much better than paper towels in draining the excess water from the tofu. It is less messy.

Low-Carb Maple Oatmeal

Serves: 1 Total Time: 25 min

Ingredients:

- ½ cup of walnuts
- ½ cup of pecans
- ¼ cup of sunflower seeds
- ¼ cup of coconut flakes
- 1000 ml. of almond milk, unsweetened
- 3/8 tsp. of stevia powder
- ½ tsp. of cinnamon
- 4 Tbsp. of chia seeds
- 1 tsp. of maple flavoring (if desired)

Instructions:

1. Put the pecans, sunflower seeds, and walnuts in a food processor. Pulse several times, enough just to crumble them.

2. Place all the ingredients in a large-sized pot. Set on low, and allow simmering for about 20 to 30 minutes. Stir thoroughly until most of the liquids are absorbed by the chia seeds. Stirring continuously will also prevent the seeds from sticking to the bottom of the pot.
3. Once the oatmeal thickens, turn the heat off.
4. Serve and enjoy right away while still hot. Alternatively, you can allow it to cool down or chill in the refrigerator for your following day's breakfast. You can also serve the oatmeal topped with your favorite fresh fruits or other toppings.

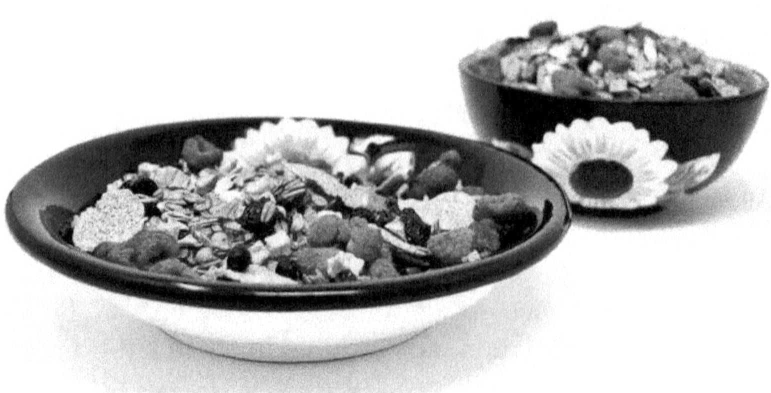

Chapter 5: Vegan Keto Lunch Recipes

Vegan Caesar Salad Quick and Easy

Serves: 4 Total Time: 5 min

Ingredients:

- 1 pc. ripe avocado
- 2 Tbsp. water
- 3 Tbsp. lemon juice
- 1 Tbsp. of caper brine
- 3 garlic cloves, minced
- 2 tsp. of Dijon mustard
- 1 Tbsp. of capers
- ¼ cup of hemp seeds
- 12 cups of romaine leaves, chopped
- Fresh ground pepper & sea salt, to taste

Instructions:

1. Put the avocado, water, lemon juice, brine, garlic, mustard, salt & pepper, and capers in the blender or food processor. Process until smooth. Add more water if you need to thin it

out a bit, depending on the size of the avocado. You should get the same consistency of a pudding if you want to keep it creamy.

2. Spoon the dressing into a small-sized bowl. Toss the hemp seeds. Stir well.
3. Put romaine in a large-sized salad bowl. Put the dressing on top. Rotate the leaves until they are completely coated.
4. Serve right away!

Low-Carb Noodle Bowls w/ Creamy Curry Sauce

Serves: 4 Total Time: 15 min

Ingredients:

For the Noodle Bowl

- 16 g of Kanten Noodles (1 pack)
- 2 pcs. of carrots, julienned
- 1 pc. of red bell pepper, diced
- ½ head of cauliflower, roughly chopped
- 2 handfuls of mixed greens
- 2 cups of water

- 1 handful of fresh cilantro, chopped

For the Creamy Curry Sauce

- 2 Tbsp. of avocado or MCT oil
- ¼ cup of tahini (substitute with avocado oil mayo, if desired)
- 2 Tbsp. of apple cider vinegar
- ¼ cup of water
- 2 tsp. of curry powder
- 1 tsp. of ground turmeric
- 1 ½ tsp. of ground coriander
- 1 tsp. of ground cumin
- 1 tsp. of sea salt
- ¼ tsp. of ground ginger
- ½ tsp. of ground black pepper

Instructions:

1. To prepare the noodles, place the noodle sheets in a large-sized bowl. Heat 2 cups of water just a little under boiling point. It should be just hot enough for you to drink. Pour the water over the noodles. Set it aside as you prepare the remaining ingredients. After soaking for around 5 minutes,

strain the noodles. Transfer to a large-sized bowl, and allow cooling.

2. Put the cauliflower, carrots, cilantro, and bell pepper into the bowl. Divide the mixed greens into 2 serving plates. This will serve as the meal's "base."
3. Put all the ingredients for the curry sauce in a blender, then process until you achieve a smooth consistency. Pour the mixture over the noodles and veggies. Toss to coat well.
4. Serve right away or refrigerate for 2 hours to allow cooling. It can last for 2 days in the refrigerator when stored in an airtight container.

Asian-Style Spiralized Zucchini Salad

Serves: 10 Total Time: 10 min

Ingredients:

- 1 pc. of medium-sized zucchini, spiralized thinly
- 1 lb. of cabbage, shredded
- 1 cup of almonds, sliced
- 1 cup of sunflower, seeds shelled
- 1/3 cup of rice vinegar or white vinegar

- ¾ cup of avocado oil
- 1 tsp. of stevia drops

Instructions:

1. Slice the zucchini into small pieces using a kitchen knife or shears. Set aside.
2. Mix the sunflower seeds, almonds, and cabbage together in a large-sized bowl. Stir the zucchini in.
3. Get a separate small-sized bowl. Mix the vinegar, oil, and stevia together using a fork or by whisking.
4. Pour the dressing over the veggies. Stir thoroughly.
5. Refrigerate for about 2 hours to chill. Serve.

Vegan Cream of Mushroom Soup

Serves: 2 Total Time: 40 min

Ingredients:

- 2 cups of cauliflower florets
- 1 tsp. of onion powder
- 1 cup of almond milk, unsweetened

- Black pepper, freshly ground, to taste
- ¼ tsp. of Himalayan rock salt
- 1 ½ cups of white mushrooms, diced
- ½ pc. of yellow onion, diced
- ½ tsp. of extra virgin olive oil

Instructions:

1. Put the milk, cauliflower, salt & pepper, and onion powder in a small-sized saucepan. Cover the pan and heat over medium setting. Bring to a boil, then lower heat. Allow simmering for about 7 to 8 minutes or until the cauliflower softens. Puree the veggies using a blender or food processor.
2. Put oil, onion, and mushrooms in a medium-sized saucepan. Cook at high heat setting until onions start to brown and become translucent or for around 8 minutes.
3. Add the pureed cauliflower mixture to the sautéed mushrooms. Cover, bring to a boil, then allow to simmer until the mixture thickens or for about 10 minutes.
4. Serve and enjoy while hot!

Creamy Roasted Red Pepper Soup

Serves: 4 Total Time: 30 min

Ingredients:

- 2 Tbsp. of coconut oil, unrefined
- 1 pc. of large-sized shallot, chopped finely
- ½ cup of roasted red pepper, chopped
- 1 tsp. of paprika
- 1 pinch of red pepper flakes, crushed
- 1 Tbsp. of seasoned salt
- 1 tsp. of sea salt
- 5 cups of cauliflower florets
- 4 cups of vegetable stock
- 1 cup of coconut milk
- 1 splash of apple cider vinegar
- 1 pinch of fresh thyme

Instructions:

1. Heat coconut oil in a heavy-bottomed pot or Dutch oven at medium heat setting.
2. Sauté shallots until they become translucent and soft, or around three minutes. Toss in the roasted peppers and seasonings, and then stir thoroughly to combine well. Cook for around 2 to 3 minutes.
3. Add stock, cauliflower, thyme, and vinegar. Once it simmers, cover the pot. Allow to cook for another 10 to 15 minutes or until cauliflower softens and starts to fall apart.
4. Working carefully in small batches, puree the soup in your blender until smooth. Bring the well-blended soup back on the stove. Slowly mix the coconut milk in.

Tempeh, Broccoli, Olives, and Spinach

Serves: 1 Total Time: 10 min

Ingredients:

- 1 cup of frozen spinach
- 1 cup of broccoli florets
- 3 oz. of tempeh, chopped
- 6 pcs. of large-sized olives

- Olive oil, garlic powder, and salt & pepper to garnish

Instructions:

1. Heat some oil in a pan. Sauté all vegetables at low heat setting, and allow to cook until done.
2. Drizzle with preferred seasonings.
3. Serve and enjoy while hot.

Kelp Noodles w/ Avocado Pesto

Serves: 4 Total Time: 45 min

Ingredients:

For the Noodles

- 1 pack of kelp noodles

For the Pesto:

- 1 pc. of Hass avocado
- 1 cup of fresh baby spinach leaves
- ½ cup of extra virgin oil
- ¼ cup of fresh basil
- 2 cloves of garlic

- 1 tsp. of salt

Instructions:

1. Rinse kelp noodles thoroughly. Soak in water for 30 minutes or more. After soaking for a few minutes, break the noodles apart from the clump. By this time, the noodles become more manageable and easier to soak.
2. Leave the noodles while they are soaking. Meanwhile, combine all pesto ingredients in a food processor or blender. Blitz until you achieve a smooth consistency. Depending on your preference, you may leave small pieces of leaves or you may process until everything is well-blended.
3. Drain the noodles after 30 minutes. Add ¼ cup of pesto for each bag of noodles.
4. Mix the noodles with the pesto thoroughly. Top with your favorite toppings.
5. Serve and enjoy!

Low-Carb Bibimbap, Vegan Version

Serves: 2 Total Time: 25 min

Ingredients:

- 200 g of tempeh, cut into small squares
- 6 pcs. of broccoli florets (thin spears)
- 2 Tbsp. of rice vinegar (substitute with regular white vinegar, if preferred)
- 1 Tbsp. of soy sauce
- ½ pc. of cucumber, cut in strips
- 1 pc. of small-sized red bell pepper, cut in strips
- 1 pc. of carrot, grated
- 300 g. of raw cauliflower, riced
- 2 Tbsp. of rice vinegar
- 2 Tbsp. of sesame seeds
- 1 tsp. of sesame oil
- 1 Tbsp. of soy sauce

- Liquid sweetener (concentrated), to taste

Instructions:

1. Combine the soy sauce and vinegar in a medium-sized bowl. Dip the tempeh squares in the mixture. Set aside for 1 or 2 minutes. Meanwhile, cut the veggies.
2. Heat some oil in a skillet. Fry the tempeh over medium heat setting. Once done, remove the tempeh from the pan. Sauté the broccoli, carrot, and peppers on the same pan. Cover the pan, and allow cooking for 1 or 2 minutes more to allow the vegetables to retain their bite.
3. In a separate pan, heat some oil, and then stir fry cauliflower rice until it becomes tender.
4. Get a small-sized bowl. Combine the vinegar, soy sauce, chili paste, sweetener, and oil. Put some water if you find the sauce too thick. Halve the cauliflower rice and place on two plates. Top each plate with tempeh, broccoli, carrot, pepper, and raw cucumber. Pour chili sauce on top of the tempeh and veggies. Sprinkle sesame seeds on top. Mix everything well on your plate before you dig in. Enjoy!

Shirataki Noodles w/ Sauce, Veggies & "Beyond Meat

Serves: 1   Total Time: 10 min

Ingredients:

- 1 pack of shirataki noodles, drained and rinsed thoroughly (if preferred, substitute with kelp)
- ½ cup of marinara sauce
- ½ cup of mixed vegetables
- 1 serving of Beyond Meat "chicken strips"

Instructions:

1. Heat some oil in a pan. Sauté all vegetables at low heat setting, and allow to cook until done.
2. Drizzle with preferred seasonings.
3. Serve and enjoy while hot.

One-Pot Zucchini Pasta

Serves: 4 Total Time: 20 min

Ingredients:

- 2 lbs. of zucchini, spiralized
- 1 pint of cherry tomatoes, cut in halves
- 4 cloves of garlic, minced
- 1 large-sized red onion, sliced thinly
- ½ cup of fresh basil
- ¼ cup of extra virgin olive oil
- ½ tsp. of red pepper, crushed (if preferred)
- Parmesan cheese, for topping, shredded (if preferred)
- Salt & pepper, for seasoning

Instructions:

1. Warm olive oil in a large-sized pot at low to medium heat setting. Put the onion and garlic, cook for about 3 minutes or until fragrant.

2. Add the noodles. Season with some salt & pepper. Place the pot cover on. Allow cooking for about 2 minutes. Stir halfway through the cooking time.

3. Put the tomatoes into the pot. Continue cooking for 3 to 4 minutes more. Stir every 30 seconds. You may use tongs for tossing the needles. This will help make sure the noodles cook evenly, and still a bit firm. To test for doneness, get a piece of the noodle to check if it is tender enough for you. If it is not, continue cooking for a few minutes more until you achieve your desired level of doneness.

4. Add the red pepper, basil, and Parmesan cheese to the dish. Stir everything well. Prepare two plates and divide the pasta equally between them. Garnish each plate with fresh basil. Serve and enjoy while still warm!

**Note: If there are leftovers, store them in airtight containers for as long as 2 days. The zucchini may produce some water while it sits. You can just drain it before you reheat.

Harissa Portobello Mushroom Tacos

Serves: 6 tacos (1 taco/serving)   Total Time: 20 mins

Ingredients:

For the Portobello Mushrooms

- 1 lb. of Portobello mushrooms
- ¼ cup of spicy harissa (use mild harissa, if you prefer it less spicy)
- 1 tsp. of ground cumin
- 3 Tbsp. of olive oil, divided
- 6 pcs. of collard green leaves
- 1 tsp. of onion powder

For the Guacamole

- 2 pcs. of medium-sized ripe avocados
- 2 Tbsp. of red onions, chopped
- 2 Tbsp. of tomatoes, chopped

- 2 Tbsp. of lemon juice (use lime juice, instead if preferred)
- 1 Tbsp. of cilantro, chopped
- 1 pinch of salt

For the Toppings (only if preferred)

- Chopped tomatoes
- Chopped cilantro
- Cashew cream

Instructions:

1. Remove the Portobello stems. Rinse the mushrooms well, and then pat to dry.
2. Combine the harissa, cumin, olive oil, onion powder in a large-sized bowl. Brush each of the mushrooms with the harissa mix. Make sure that the mushroom edges are covered as well. Allow the mushroom to marinate for about 15 minutes.
3. While marinating the mushrooms, prepare the guacamole. Cut the avocadoes in halves, and then pit them. Mash the avocadoes, and then add the red onions, tomatoes, cilantro, lemon juice, and salt. Mix well, and then set aside.
4. Rinse the collard greens well. Chop the tough stems off, and then set aside.

5. Once the mushrooms have been marinated, heat some olive oil in a sauté pan or skillet at medium-high heat setting. Put the mushrooms in the heated pan, and allow cooking for about 3 minutes. After 3 minutes, flip the mushrooms over, and allow cooking for 3 minutes more. Make sure that each of the sides is browned.

6. Turn the heat off. Allow the mushrooms to rest for about 3 minutes first before slicing.

7. Take a piece of collard green leaf. Fill it with several slices of Portobello mushroom. Top with cashew cream, cilantro, and chopped tomatoes as desired.

8. Serve and enjoy!

**Notes: If you want to make cashew cream on your own, soak a cup of raw cashews and leave it overnight. Drain the water, and then blend the cashews with a fresh cup of water. You can use the cream on the tacos or consume it as is. Just season with some salt and lemon juice.

When using very thick harissa, you can blend it with some oil. Then, add a Tbsp. of water at a time to help thin it out. Make sure that you adjust the seasonings as well.

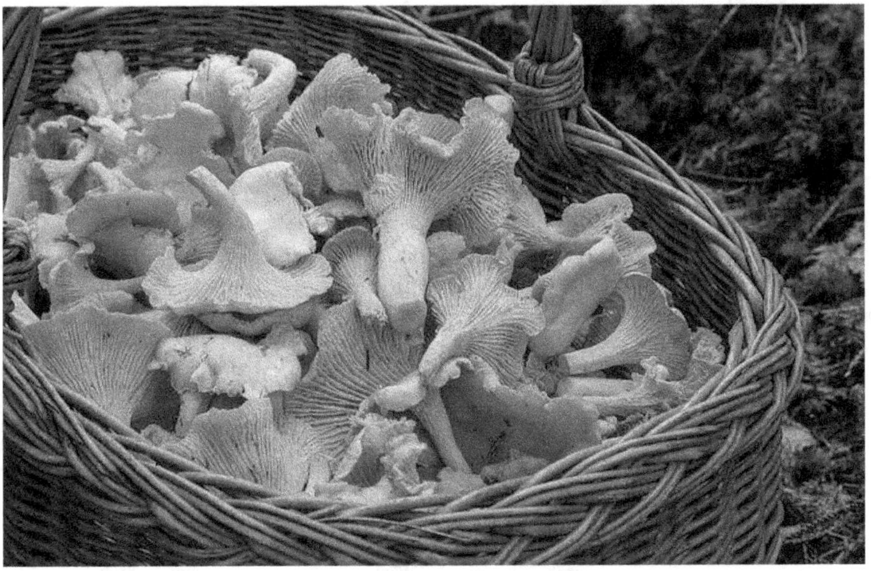

Brussels Sprouts, Hummus, and Spinach

Serves: 1 Total Time: 10 min

Ingredients:

- 1 cup of Brussels sprouts, chopped
- 4 Tbsp. of hummus
- 1 cup of frozen spinach
- Olive oil, garlic powder, and salt & pepper to garnish

Instructions:

1. Heat some oil in a pan. Sauté all vegetables at low heat setting, and allow to cook until done.
2. Drizzle with preferred seasonings.
3. Serve and enjoy while hot.

Thai-Style Roasted Cauliflower Soup

Serves: 6 Total Time: 40 min

Ingredients:

- 1 pc. large-sized cauliflower
- 1 pc. of medium-sized yellow onion, diced
- 4 cups of veggie broth
- 5 Tbsp. of Thai red curry paste
- 1 Tbsp. of olive oil
- 14 oz. of unsweetened coconut milk
- 1 Tbsp. of lemon juice
- ¼ tsp. of Himalayan pink salt
- Green onions, for garnish

Instructions:

1. Pre-heat oven to 400° F.
2. Cut off the cauliflower florets. Cut the onion into 4 quarters. Lay down the cauliflower and onion cuts on a baking tray w/ parchment paper lining. Add olive oil and allow baking for about 20 minutes.
3. Put the roasted veggies and vegetable broth in a blender, and process until the mixture is completely smooth and creamy.
4. Pour the puree into a medium-sized soup pot. Heat over medium setting. Add the coconut milk, lemon juice, salt, and red curry paste. Stir well. Allow cooking until the dish is hot all over.
5. Pour soup into separate bowls, and garnish with green onions.
6. Serve and enjoy while hot!

Fast and Easy Vegan Cauliflower Rice

Serves: 1 Total Time: 10 min

Ingredients:

- 1 cup of cauliflower florets
- Your favorite vegan toppings

Instructions:

1. Cut the cauliflower florets off.
2. Put the cauliflower florets in a food processor or blender. Process until the veggie looks like small rice granules.
3. Sauté for a couple of minutes or until warm.
4. Top with your favorite vegan toppings.
5. Serve and enjoy right away!

Broccoli Fried Rice

Serves: 4 Total Time: 8 min

Ingredients:

- 4 cups of riced broccoli
- 1 Tbsp. of garlic, finely chopped
- 1 Tbsp. of avocado oil
- 1 ½ tsp. of sesame oil
- 1 Tbsp. of coconut oil
- ½ tsp. of coarse salt, to taste
- Juice of 1 quarter of a lemon (more if desired)
- 2 bulbs of scallions, chopped
- 4 tbsp. of cilantro or parsley, chopped (if preferred)

Instructions:

1. Heat a tsp. of oil in a skillet. Sauté the broccoli rice with garlic for about 1 minute. Season with toasted sesame oil, coarse salt, and coconut aminos. Sauté for two minutes more. Make sure to cook the broccoli until it achieves a bright green color, retaining some bite. It must not be mushy.

2. Put the heat off. While the "rice" is still warm, roughly grate ½ tsp. of frozen ginger. Sprinkle over the rice. Drizzle with lime juice.
3. Garnish with your preferred toppings.
4. Serve and enjoy right away!

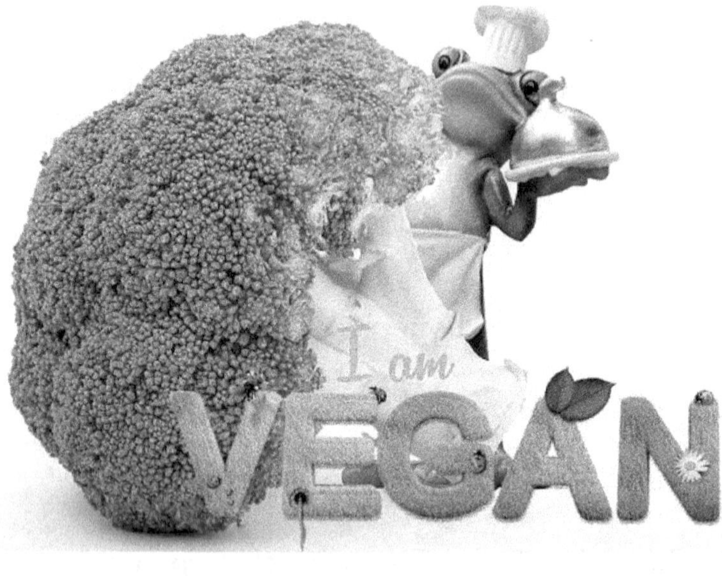

Chapter 6: Vegan Keto Dinner Recipes

Stir-Fried Beyond Meat Beef Taco

Serves: 4 Total Time: 10 min

Ingredients:

- 1 pack of cauliflower rice
- 1 pack of Beyond Meat beef crumbles
- Guacamole and some sliced olives, for toppings

Instructions:

1. Heat oil in a pan over low heat setting.
2. Combine everything in the pan, except for the toppings. Allow cooking until the cauliflower rice becomes soft.
3. Top with the guacamole and sliced olives, if desired.
4. Serve and enjoy right away!

Vegan Keto Carbonara

Serves: 1 Total Time: 40 min

Ingredients:

For the Tofu, (this makes 4 servings, so you can just keep the leftovers for later use)

- 1 block (about 400 g/14 oz.) of firm tofu
- 2 Tbsp. of olive oil
- 3 Tbsp. of low-sodium tamari
- ¼ tsp. of smoked sea salt

For the Sauce (this makes 5 servings)

- 1 cup of hulled hemp seeds
- ¼ tsp. of salt
- ¾ cup of nutritional yeast
- ¾ cup of water

For the Entire Dish

- 1 pack of shirataki noodles
- ¼ batch of the tofu mentioned above

- 1/3 cup of the above-mentioned sauce
- 1 tsp. of nutritional yeast, for serving
- 1 stalk of scallion, sliced
- 1 pinch of fresh black pepper

Instructions:

1. To prepare the tofu bacon:

   Pre-heat oven to 375° F. Line a baking sheet (rimmed) w/ parchment paper.

   Drain the tofu block, and then cut in thin slices.

   Press out the water from the tofu slices using a clean dishtowel.

   Whisk the olive oil, smoked sea salt, and tamari together in a small-sized mixing bowl.

   Dip the tofu pieces in the marinade. Then lay them down on the baking sheet.

   Pour the leftover marinade, if any over the tofu slices. Allow baking for about 30 minutes or until crispy.

2. To make the carbonara sauce:

   Put the sauce ingredients into a blender. Process thoroughly until everything is smooth, or for about 3 minutes.

3. To assemble the carbonara dish:

   Drain the noodles, then rinse well. Place them in a small-sized pan and cook at medium-low heat setting.

   Pour 1/3 of the sauce into the noodles. Stir well until noodles are coated thoroughly.

   Allow to cooking for 5 to 10 minutes or until the sauce thickens, and the extra moisture evaporates out of the noodles.

   Get ¼ of the "bacon" slices and chop into smaller pieces. Stir the bacon pieces into the noodles.

   Prepare a serving plate. If desired, sprinkle with additional nutritional yeast, fresh pepper, and scallions.

4. Serve and enjoy warm!

**Notes: In case you do not enjoy the texture or taste of shirataki noodles, you can instead use edamame noodles, zucchini noodles, or any other low-carb pasta you prefer.

Vegan Keto Bibimbap

Serves: 1 Total Time: 40 min

Ingredients:

- 1 cup of cauliflower rice, cooked
- 3.5 oz. of air-fried or baked tofu
- ½ cup of broccoli, cooked
- 1/8 cup of shiitake mushrooms, cooked
- 1 tsp. of sesame seeds
- 1 Tbsp. of low-carb gochujang
- Chopped scallions, for garnishing

Instructions:

1. Reheat veggies and cauliflower rice, if necessary, on the stovetop. Air-fry or bake the tofu for about 20 minutes or until crispy.
2. Mix the tofu with all the veggies in a medium-sized mixing bowl. Stir the gochujang in. Garnish with scallions and sesame seeds, or as desired.

3. Serve. Mix everything well before eating. Enjoy!

Mustard Dill Zucchini Cakes

Serves: 2 (2 cakes/serving) Total Time: 50 min

Ingredients:

- 12 oz. of grated zucchini (replace with summer squash, if desired)
- 1 Tbsp. of fresh dill, chopped
- 1 Tbsp. of prepared mustard
- 1 Tbsp. of extra virgin olive oil
- ½ tsp. of salt
- ¼ tsp. of granulated garlic
- ¼ cup of protein powder (you can instead use chickpea/soy/lupini flour if preferred)

Instructions:

1. Combine the grated zucchini and salt together in a medium-sized mixing bowl. Allow sitting for around 20 minutes. Press the excess moisture out using a spoon, and drain the liquid.

2. Pre-heat oven to 350° F. Line a baking sheet (rimmed) w/ parchment paper.
3. Thoroughly stir the oil, dill, garlic, and mustard into the zucchini mix until everything is combined well.
4. Add the protein powder. Equally, divide the dough into 4 portions.
5. Make 4 patties on the parchment paper-lined baking sheet. Flatten the patties to about ½".
6. Allow to bake for 30 to 40 minutes or until both sides are golden brown. Make sure to flip halfway through to ensure even cooking.
7. Take the cakes out of the oven. Allow cooking for a couple of minutes.
8. Serve and enjoy!

Vegan Keto Sushi Bowl

Serves: 1 Total Time: 5 min

Ingredients:

- ½ cup of cooked cauliflower rice

- ¼ cup of cucumber, cubed or sliced
- 1 serving of seaweed salad
- 1/3 can of Vegan Toona or any preferred protein (edamame, tofu, etc.)

For the Toppings

- ¼ pc. of avocado, sliced
- 1 tsp. of sesame seeds
- Some microgreens for sprinkling

Instructions:

1. Mix all the ingredients together in a medium-sized bowl.
2. Sprinkle the toppings.
3. Serve and enjoy right away!

Vegan Mushroom Burgers

Serves: 3 Total Time: 40 min

Ingredients:

- 8 oz. of mushrooms, sliced
- 1 Tbsp. of ground chia seeds

- ¼ cup of tahini
- ¼ tsp. of black pepper, cracked
- ½ tsp. of smoked sea salt
- ¼ tsp. of dried rosemary, ground (you can instead of your preferred seasoning)
- 3 Tbsp. of unflavoured pea protein

Instructions:

1. Pre-heat oven to 350° F. Line a baking sheet (rimmed) w/ parchment paper.
2. Cook mushrooms in a large-sized skillet at medium-low heat setting until they become completely tender. Make sure to stir often.
3. Allow cooling for a couple of minutes. Drain the excess liquid off. Chop the mushrooms roughly either by hand or using a blender or food processor.
4. Thoroughly stir in the chia seeds, tahini, rosemary, and salt & pepper with the mushrooms until everything is well combined.
5. Set the mixture aside for about 5 minutes to allow the chia seeds to absorb the excess moisture. This will also help the mixture thicken.

6. Add the protein powder until it is absorbed completely. Begin with 2 Tbsp., and then add a tsp. at a time. You want to avoid drying up the mixture. You need to stop adding protein powder when it starts not to mix in thoroughly.
7. Divide the mixture into 3 equal-sized patties. Each patty should be around 4" in diameter, and ½" thick. Lay the patties down on the baking sheet. Do not bother too much about the spacing. Allow baking for 20 to 25 minutes or until they become firm. Flip the patties after 15 minutes to ensure even cooking.
8. Take the patties out of the oven. Allow cooking for several minutes.
9. Serve and enjoy while warm!

Spaghetti Squash & Pesto

Serves: 1 Total Time: 10 min

Ingredients:

- 1 cup of spaghetti squash
- ¼ cup of pesto

- Red pepper flakes, if preferred
- Olive oil, garlic powder, and salt & pepper to garnish

Instructions:

1. Roast the squash a bit ahead of time.
2. Scoop the squash into a medium-sized bowl. Pour the pesto on top.
3. Drizzle with your preferred seasonings.
4. Serve and enjoy while hot.

Cauliflower Pizza Crust, Low-Carb Vegan-Style

Serves: 4 Total Time: 50 min

Ingredients:

- 12 oz. of cauliflower, riced
- ¼ cup of whole psyllium husk
- ¼ cup of tahini
- ¼ tsp. of salt

Instructions:

1. Pre-heat oven to 350° F. Line a baking sheet (rimmed) w/ parchment paper.
2. Cook the riced cauliflower in a medium-sized pan over medium-low heat setting. Allow cooking until the cauliflower is tender.
3. Allow to slightly cool down, then mix with the rest of the ingredients until you form a uniform dough.
4. Divide the dough equally into 2 portions. (Do not divide it if you prefer to make 1 big dough.) Roll the 2 pcs. Of dough into rounds of around ¼" thick.
5. Put the dough in the oven, and allow baking for about 15 minutes. Carefully flip the dough and bring them back to the oven to cook for another 10 to 15 minutes or until the crust turns golden brown.
6. Take the crust out of the oven. Top with your desired toppings.
7. Serve and enjoy!

Shirataki Noodles w/ Sauce, Olives, and Spinach

Serves: 1 Total Time: 10 min

Ingredients:

- 1 pack of shirataki noodles, well-drained, and rinsed
- 1 cup of frozen spinach
- ¼ cup of marinara sauce (replace with salsa, if preferred)
- 10 pcs. of small olives, sliced

Instructions:

1. Cook noodles following instructions on the package.
2. Sauté the vegetables in a pan over low heat setting until they are tender and done.
3. Pour the veggies over the cooked noodles.
4. Drizzle with your preferred seasonings.
5. Serve and enjoy while hot.

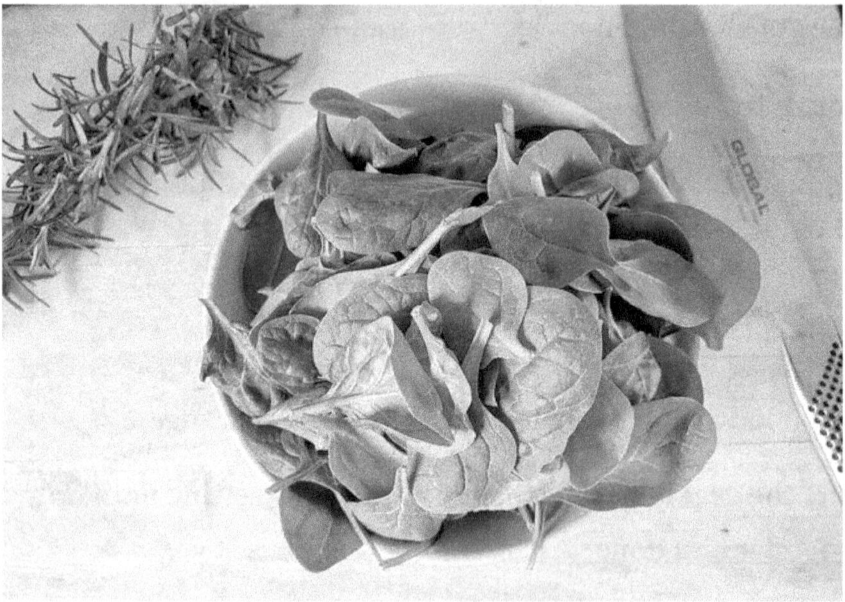

Shirataki Alfredo w/ Spinach

Serves: 1 Total Time: 10 min

Ingredients:

- 1 pack of shirataki noodles, well-drained, and rinsed
- 1 cup of frozen spinach
- 2 oz. of vegan cream cheese
- Olive oil, garlic powder, and salt & pepper to garnish

Instructions:

1. Combine all the ingredients in a pan and cook under low heat setting.
2. Stir well until you achieve your desired texture. You can add some water or milk while stirring if you prefer. If you happen to add a bit too much liquid, just allow cooking some more until the sauce becomes thicker.
3. Serve and enjoy while hot!

Stir Fry Tofu & Tomato

Serves: 1 Total Time: 9 min

Ingredients:

- 2 stalks of scallions, sliced
- 1 Tbsp. of low-sodium tamari
- 1 Tbsp. of olive oil (replace with sesame oil, if you prefer more flavor)
- ½ cup of tomatoes, sliced

- ¼ block of firm tofu
- ½ cup of cauliflower rice, cooked
- 1 pinch of salt & pepper

Instructions:

1. Heat tamari and oil in a small-sized pan over medium-low heat setting. Toss the scallions and tomatoes in. You may reserve some scallions for garnish if you prefer.
2. Stir everything well. Put the pan cover on so as not to let all the liquid to evaporate. Allow to cook for about 5 minutes, or until the tomatoes are tender.
3. Crumble the tofu into the pan. Thoroughly stir everything around. Make sure the tofu is well-coated in the tamari mixture. Cook uncovered for about 2 minutes or until you are sure the tofu is all warmed through, and all the excess liquid has evaporated or has been absorbed.
4. Take the dish away from the heat, and season with some salt & pepper, as well as the reserved scallions.
5. Serve hot over cauliflower rice. Enjoy!

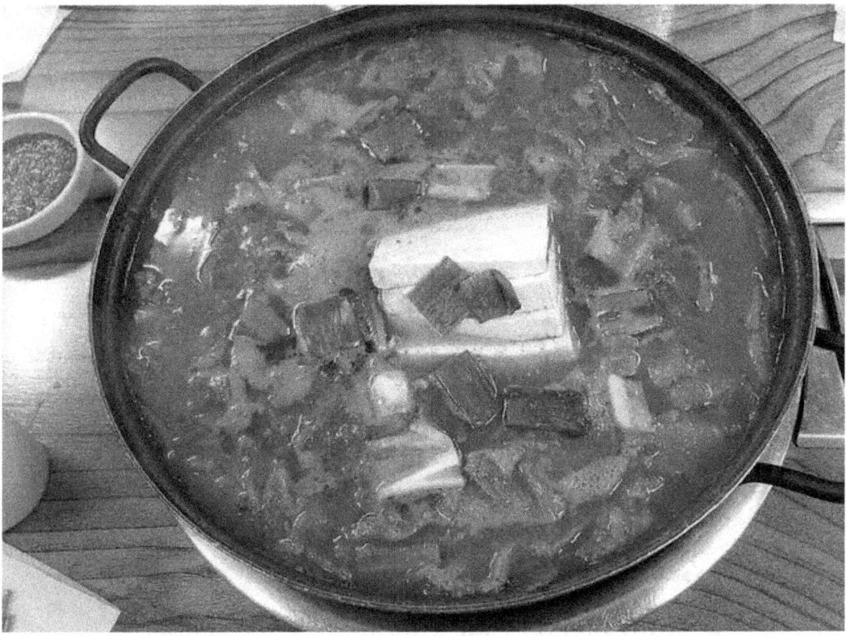

Cold Peanut Ginger Noodle Salad

Serves: 2 Total Time: 5 min

Ingredients:

- ¼ cup of unsweetened peanut butter
- 1 Tbsp. of low-sodium tamari
- ¼ cup of water
- 1 tsp. of fresh ginger, grated

- 1 clove of garlic, crushed
- 2 pcs of medium-sized zucchini noodles

For Garnishing (optional)

- Red pepper flakes
- Chopped peanuts
- Scallions

Instructions:

1. Whisk the water, peanut butter, ginger, garlic, and tamari together in a small-sized bowl. If you think the sauce is unnecessarily thick, just continue adding water a Tbsp. at a time. Stop when you achieve your desired texture.
2. Toss the sauce into the noodles. Mix well until the noodles are completely coated in sauce.
3. Pour noodles into a serving bowl. Garnish, as preferred.
4. Enjoy right away!

Sloppy Joes, Vegan Keto Version

Serves: 6 Total Time: 50 min

Ingredients:

- 1 cup of hulled pumpkin seeds (pepitas)
- ½ cup of hulled hemp seeds
- 1 cup of walnuts, chopped
- 6 oz. of tomato paste
- 1 tsp. of onion powder
- ½ Tbsp. of garlic powder
- 1 Tbsp. of apple cider vinegar
- 2 cups of veggie broth
- 1 Tbsp. of prepared mustard
- 1 Tbsp. of granulated sweetener
- Slices of bread, lettuce wraps, or rolls, for serving

Instructions:

1. Combine all ingredients in a Dutch oven or pot. Heat at medium-low setting. Cover and allow cooking for around 45 minutes, stirring from time to time, until the veggie broth is absorbed completely. Make sure to check on the mixture from time to time. Make sure that it only simmers and it does not burn.
2. Best served on keto bread or rolls. Enjoy!

Triple Green Kale Salad

Serves: 2 Total Time: 10 mins

Ingredients:

Part 1:

- 10 oz. of Lacinato or Tuscan kale, sliced into small pieces (see step 1 of instructions)
- 2 tsp. of extra virgin oil (or flaxseed oil, if preferred)
- 2 tsp. of sesame oil, toasted
- 2 cloves of small-sized garlic, crushed or grated
- 1 tsp. of fresh ginger, grated
- 1 pinch of sea salt, coarse

Part 2:

- 1 handful of snow peas, chopped
- 2 tsp. of balsamic vinegar, aged
- 2 tsp. of coconut aminos
- 1 pc. of ripe avocado, sliced
- 1 handful of scallions, chopped

- Zest of orange
- Hemp seeds for sprinkling

Instructions:

1. Thoroughly was the kale and rinse well. Pat to dry. Lay a leaf of kale down on a cutting board. Run a paring knife along the sides of the center stem, one side at a time. Repeat the process until you have removed all the stems. Stack about 5 layers of leaves. Roll them to facilitate slicing into small pieces.
2. Mix the chopped kale leaves with the rest of the ingredients listed under Part 1. Wash your hands thoroughly, and then massage the kale gently. Rub the oil onto the kale leaves for several seconds.
3. Add the ingredients listed under Part 2. Toss everything briskly.
4. Serve right away at room temperature. If preferred, chill slightly before serving.
5. Enjoy!

Chapter 7: Vegan Keto Dessert and Side Dish Recipes

Vegan Keto Desserts

Vegan Keto Raw Strawberry Crumble

Serves: 5 Total Time: 5 min

Ingredients:

- 1 lb. of fresh strawberries
- ½ cup of raw walnuts
- ¼ cup of dried coconut
- ½ Tbsp. of ground cinnamon
- ½ Tbsp. of grated ginger

Instructions:

1. Wash and rinse strawberries. De-stem then slices them into smaller pieces. Arrange the strawberries in a serving container like a pie dish.
2. Place the strawberries in a high-speed blender or food processor. Blitz in the rest of the ingredients until you form a crumble that is enough to hold shape when you pinch them together.

3. Garnish the dish by crumbling the toppings as desired.

4. Serve and enjoy!

Peanut Butter Chocolate Pumpkin, Vegan Keto Style

Serves: 10 (1 pumpkin/serving)   Total Time: 3 hours 30 min

Ingredients:

- ¼ cup of unsweetened peanut butter
- ¼ cup of cocoa butter
- ¼ cup of coconut milk powder, divided
- Liquid stevia, to taste (if preferred)
- 1 Tbsp. of chia seeds
- 1 tsp. of vanilla extract
- 2 Tbsp. of MCT oil

Instructions:

1. Stir 2 Tbsp. of coconut milk powder together with the chia seeds and peanut butter. If you prefer using sweetener, stir in the stevia.

2. Roll the "dough" into small balls. If it is not firm enough, refrigerate it for a few hours to chill until it becomes firm.

3. Make 10 equal-sized balls from the dough. Flatten each one into discs. Each disc should be around ½ Tbsp. and measure about 1" in diameter and 1/3" tall.

4. Chill the balls for around 15 to 20 minutes to make them firmer.

5. Melt the oils together. Once completely melted, add 2 Tbsp. of coconut milk powder plus the vanilla extract. Thoroughly stir to combine well.

6. Get a silicon mold, and put about 1 tsp. of the cocoa butter mix on each cavity. Fill up 10 cavities. What you want is to evenly cover the bottom.

7. Allow the partially-filled old to freeze until some of the cocoa butter blends is completely chilled. This should take as long as the time it would take the peanut butter discs to harden.

8. Remove the peanut butter discs from the freezer. Put a disc in each cavity, making sure that it is on top of the layer of cocoa butter.

9. Stir in the rest of the cocoa butter mixture, making sure it combines well. Evenly distribute it on top of each peanut butter disc. Ideally, the top and all sides of the discs. It is no

big deal, though if they are not completely covered. Just make sure the sides are covered.

10. Chill in the refrigerator for no less than 3 hours or until everything is completely hard.
11. Serve chilled and enjoy!

Strawberry and Nuts Crumble

Serves: 5 Total Time: 5 min

Ingredients:

- 1 lb. of fresh strawberries
- ½ cup of raw walnuts
- ¼ cup of macadamia nuts (or another fatty nut like Brazil nuts, walnuts, or pecans)
- ½ Tbsp. of ground cinnamon
- ½ Tbsp. of grated ginger

Instructions:

1. Wash and rinse strawberries. De-stem then slices them into smaller pieces. Arrange the strawberries in a serving container like a pie dish.

2. Place the strawberries in a high-speed blender or food processor. Blitz in the rest of the ingredients until you form a crumble that is enough to hold shape when you pinch them together.
3. Garnish the dish by crumbling the toppings as desired.
4. Serve and enjoy!

Chocolate Hazelnut Spread

Serves: 16 (2 Tbsp. each serving) Total Time: 5 min

Ingredients:

- 1 cup of sunflower seeds
- 1 ½ cups of hazelnuts
- ½ cup of desiccated coconut
- ½ cup of MCT oil
- 3 Tbsp. of cacao powder
- 1 pinch of salt
- 15 drops of stevia to taste

Instructions:

1. Place the sunflower seeds, hazelnuts, oil, and coconut. Process until you achieve a liquid and smooth consistency or about 3 minutes. You can start processing at level 1, gradually increasing the speed every 15 seconds or as the nut butter gets smoother.
2. Add 1 Tbsp. of cocoa powder at a time, completely blending before adding the next teaspoon. This will help you reach a smooth consistency without the powder having to explode back up.
3. Add the salt and sweetener, as you prefer. Add more or less, depending on the level of sweetness you want.
4. To serve, spread on a slice of toast or drizzle over ice cream or by itself on a spoon.

Vegan Keto No-Bake Lemon Squares

Serves: 8 squares (1 square each serving) Total Time: 5 min

Ingredients:

- 1 cup of dried coconut, unsweetened
- 1 cup of macadamia nuts

- ¼ cup of lemon juice
- ¼ cup of coconut oil
- 1 tsp. of vanilla extract
- 1 Tbsp. of granulated sweetener
- Lemon zest, if preferred

Instructions:

1. Line some parchment paper on a loaf pan. You can use a silicon loaf pan, instead to avoid sticking.
2. Process all ingredients in a high-speed blender or food processor until you form a smooth dough. A process on low setting for around 2 minutes, then switches to medium for 1 minute. Stop the processor every 20 seconds or so to scrape the sides. The dough should look a lot similar to cookie dough. Make sure that no pieces of coconut or nut remain.
3. Transfer the dough to the lined pan by scooping. Smoothen it. If preferred, you can top it with lemon zest. Chill it for half an hour in the freezer to allow it to set.
4. Get the bars out of the pan. Slice them into a total of 8 squares. Store in the refrigerator. Remove when ready to serve.

Red Velvet Cupcakes, Vegan Keto-Style

Serves: 4 cupcakes Total Time: 45 min

Ingredients:

For the Cupcakes:

- ¼ cup of tahini (if preferred, substitute tahini with almond butter)
- ¼ cup of coconut milk, unsweetened (or another non-dairy milk, if preferred)
- 2 Tbsp. of granulated sweetener
- 2 Tbsp. of ground flax seed
- 1 Tbsp. of apple cider vinegar
- 2 heaped Tbsp. of cocoa powder
- 1 Tbsp. of beetroot powder
- ¼ tsp. of baking soda
- ½ tsp. of baking powder

For the Frosting:

- ¼ cup of vegan cheese cream
- ¼ cup of coconut cream
- 5 drops of liquid stevia, to taste

Instructions:

1. Preheat oven to 350° F. Line the 4 wells of a regular-sized muffin pan with some paper liners. If preferred, you can instead use regular-size muffin liners or muffin pan.
2. Whisk the coconut milk, tahini, and vinegar together in a small-sized mixing bowl until thoroughly blended and smooth. Add the flax seeds and sweetener. Stir well, and then set aside.
3. Get a separate bowl, and then whisk the beetroot powder, baking soda, baking powder, and cocoa powder together thoroughly until well-combined. Smush any visible clumps using a fork.
4. Fold the dry mixture gently into the wet ingredients. Stir well until you no longer see any clumps. Avoid stirring too roughly; otherwise, you may ruin the volume from the reaction of the baking soda and vinegar together.

5. Equally, divide the batter among the 4 muffin wells lined with paper. Fill each well ¾ of the way. Allow to bake for 25 to 30 minutes, or until it becomes firm to the touch.

6. Take the dish out of the oven. Allow to cool and set while still in the pan or for about 10 minutes. Once the cupcakes have set, take them out of the pan, and allow to completely cool down before frosting.

7. To prepare the frosting, mix the coconut cream and cream cheese together. Add stevia if preferred. Stir well until you achieve a smooth consistency. Divide the frosting among the cupcakes.

Gingerbread Muffins

Serves: 5 muffins   Total Time: 50 min

Ingredients:

- ¾ cup of non-dairy milk (or water, if preferred)
- ¼ cup of granulated sweetener
- 1 Tbsp. of melted coconut oil (MCT oil can be used, instead if preferred)
- 1 tsp. of vanilla extract

- ½ cup of ground flax seeds
- 1 ½ tsp. of grated ginger (fresh or dried)
- ½ cup of coconut flour
- ¼ tsp. of ground nutmeg
- 1 ½ tsp. of ground cinnamon
- ¼ tsp. of ground allspice
- ¼ tsp. of ground cloves

Instructions:

1. Pre-heat oven to 375° F.
2. Line the 5 wells of a regular-sized muffin pan using paper liners.
3. Whisk the non-dairy milk, sweetener, flaxseeds, vanilla, and oil together. Set aside for 5 minutes to let the flax seeds to gel up.
4. Get a separate small-sized bowl. Whisk together the remaining ingredients using a dry fork.
5. Stir the dry ingredients briskly into the wet ingredients, until the mixture has thickened, and making sure that no clumps remain.

6. Scoop the batter carefully into the muffin pans lined wells. Fill each well fully. Allow baking for 30 to 35 minutes until the tops are firm when touched. To test for doneness, poke the batter with a knife. If the knife comes out clean, then it is done.
7. Remove the dish from the oven. Allow cooling while still in the pan for 15 minutes or more. Make sure that the muffins have already set before removing from the pan.
8. When the muffins have cooled down enough, they should pop out easily from the pan. When using a silicone muffin pan w/o liners, make sure to run a knife along each well's outer edge after the muffins have cooled down. This will facilitate removing the muffins from the wells.
9. Serve and enjoy right away!

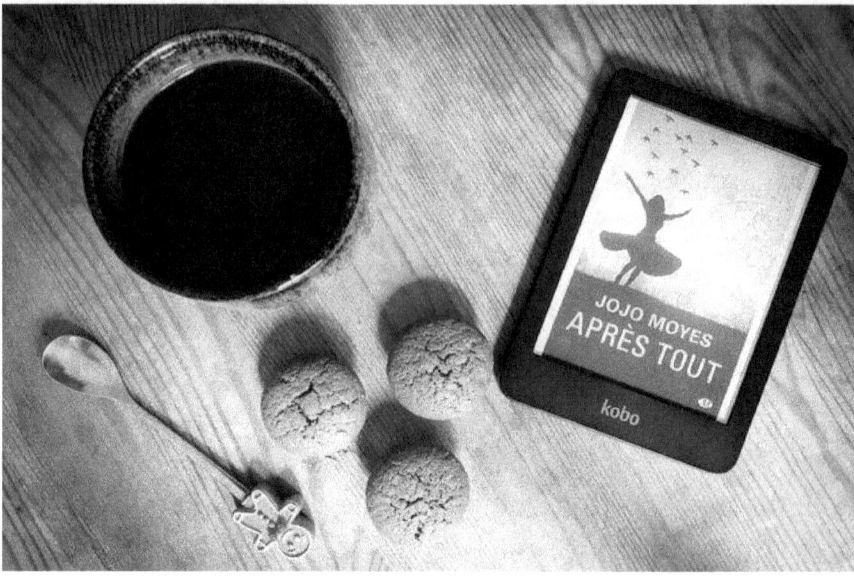

Vegan Keto Eggnog (Dairy-Free, Egg-Free Version)

Serves: 5 cups (1 cup/serving)   Total Time: 5 min

Ingredients:

- 3 cups of non-dairy milk, unsweetened (or water if preferred)
- 1 cup of pecans, raw and unsalted
- 2 Tbsp. of granulated sweetener
- 1 tsp. of vanilla extract

- ¼ cup of vanilla protein powder
- 1 tsp. of nutmeg, ground
- 1 tiny pinch of salt
- 1 pinch of cinnamon or allspice

Instructions:

1. Put all the ingredients together in a high-speed blender. Process until everything is smooth or around 1 ½ minute. Start processing at a low setting, and then switch to high setting for the final 30 seconds.
2. If you prefer super smooth eggnog, strain the beverage with the use of a nut-milk bag. Skip this step altogether if you are already satisfied with the consistency.
3. Serve and enjoy while still warm. Alternatively, you can store it in the refrigerator for a few hours if you prefer to consume your eggnog chilled. Just warm up some eggnog on the stove if you want it hot.

Strawberry Lemon Crumble

Serves: 5 Total Time: 5 min

Ingredients:

- 1 lb. of fresh strawberries
- ½ cup of raw walnuts
- ¼ cup of dried coconut
- 1 Tbsp. of lemon zest
- ½ Tbsp. of grated ginger

Instructions:

1. Wash and rinse strawberries. De-stem then slices them into smaller pieces. Arrange the strawberries in a serving container like a pie dish.
2. Place the strawberries in a high-speed blender or food processor. Blitz in the rest of the ingredients until you form a crumble that is enough to hold shape when you pinch them together.
3. Garnish the dish by crumbling the toppings as desired.
4. Serve and enjoy!

Chocolate Almond Butter Cupcakes

Serves: 4 (1 cupcake/serving) Total Time: 45 min

Ingredients:

- ¼ cup of unsweetened creamy almond butter kept at room temperature
- ¼ cup of unsweetened almond milk, or any preferred non-dairy milk
- 2 Tbsp. of ground flax seeds
- 2 Tbsp. of granulated sweetener
- ½ tsp. of baking powder
- 2 Tbsp. of cocoa powder

For the Frosting:

- 2 Tbsp. of vegan keto cream cheese
- 1 Tbsp. of creamy almond butter, unsweetened
- 2 Tbsp. of unsweetened almond milk
- Stevia sweetener, if preferred

Instructions:

1. Pre-heat oven to 350° F.
2. Line 4 of the wells of a regular-sized muffin pan using paper liners.
3. Mix the almond milk and almond butter together in a small-sized mixing bowl. Whisk thoroughly until smooth and well-

combined. Add the flax seeds and sweetener. Stir well, and then set aside.

4. Mix the baking powder and cocoa powder together in a separate mixing bowl. Whisk thoroughly with a dry fork until everything is well-combined.
5. Fold dry ingredients gently into the wet ingredients. Continue stirring until there are no remaining lumps.
6. Evenly divide the batter among the 4 muffin wells. Fill each well ¾ full. Allow to bake for about 30 minutes or until the batter feels firm when touched.
7. Take the dish out of the oven. Allow the muffins to cool while still in the pan or for about 20 minutes. Remove the muffins from the pan. Set aside to allow to completely cool down before frosting.
8. For the frosting, put cream in a small-sized mixing bowl. Add the almond milk, almond butter, and your preferred flavoring.
9. Serve right away!

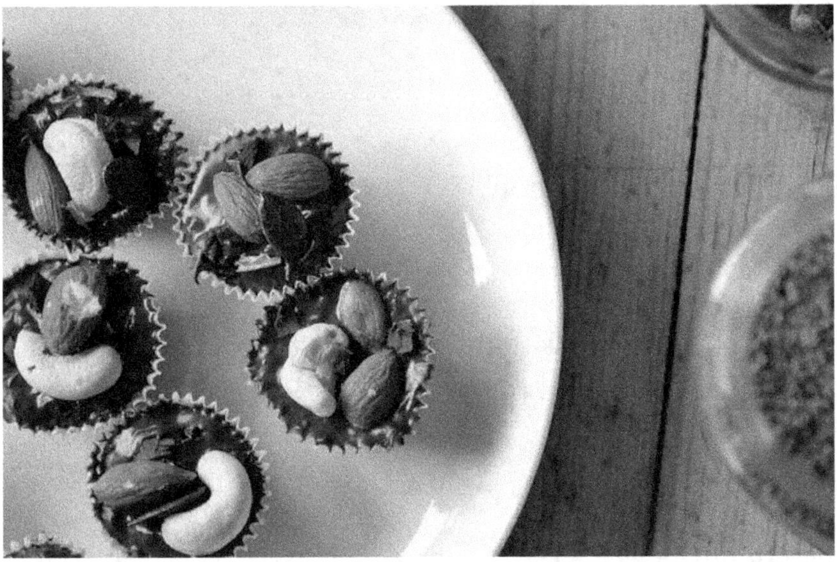

Vegan Keto-Style Cider Doughnuts

Serves: 6 (1 doughnut/serving)   Total Time: 45 min

Ingredients:

Wet Ingredients:

- ½ cup + 2 Tbsp. of non-dairy milk (replace with water, if preferred)
- ½ cup of coconut manna
- 3 Tbsp. of granulated sweetener
- 1 tsp. of vanilla extract
- 1 Tbsp. of apple cider vinegar

Dry Ingredients:

- 3 Tbsp. of coconut flour
- ¼ tsp. of ground cinnamon
- ¼ tsp. of baking powder
- 1 Tbsp. of psyllium husk (substitute w/ 1 tsp. of psyllium husk powder, if preferred)
- 1 pinch of salt
- 1 pinch of nutmeg

Instructions:

1. Pre-heat oven to 350° F. Grease a regular-sized doughnut pan.
2. Put the wet ingredients together in a double boiler and whisk until evenly mixed and melted, or for about 5 minutes.
3. While heating the wet ingredients, transfer the dry ingredients into a small-sized mixing bowl, and whisk thoroughly using a clean fork.
4. When the wet ingredients are all melted and combined, take the bowl away from the double boiler. Completely stir the dry ingredients in. Allow the mixture to sit for about 5 minutes to allow the psyllium to gel up.

5. Distribute the batter evenly into 6 of the doughnut pan's cavities. Smooth out the top.
6. Allow to bake for 25 to 30 minutes or until the edges turn golden. To test for doneness, insert a toothpick in the thickest part of the dough. Cooking is done when it comes out clean.
7. Take the doughnuts out of the oven. Allow to completely cool, and then remove from the pan.
8. Serve and enjoy right away!

Vegan Keto-Style Chocolate Doughnuts

Serves: 6 (1 doughnut/serving)   Total Time: 30 min

Ingredients:

Dry Ingredients:

- 3 Tbsp. of psyllium husk (if preferred, substitute w/ 2 tsp. of psyllium husk powder)
- 3 Tbsp. of cocoa powder (not rounded, but scooped and flattened)
- 1 pinch of salt

Wet Ingredients:

- ½ cup of tahini
- ½ cup of brewed coffee (if preferred, replace with non-dairy milk)
- ½ tsp. of baking powder
- 1 tsp. of vanilla extract
- 3 Tbsp. of granulated sweetener

Instructions:

1. Pre-heat oven to 350° F. has a greased standard-sized doughnut pan ready.
2. Whisk together the dry ingredients in a small-sized bowl. Set aside.
3. Mix all the wet ingredients together in a medium-sized mixing bowl. Stir thoroughly until everything is combined well.
4. Stir in the dry ingredients until they form a thick batter. Allow it to sit for about 3 to 5 minutes. This will give the batter enough time to thicken.
5. Distribute the batter evenly in the doughnut pan. Smoothen any large peaks.
6. Place the pan in the oven. Bake for about 25 minutes or until the top parts firm up, and the edges turn golden in color.

Remove the pan from heat and allow the doughnuts to cool down for around 10 minutes while still in the pan.

7. Remove the doughnuts from the pan only once they have set.
8. Serve and enjoy!

Vegan Keto Side Dishes

Vegan Keto Crack Slaw

Serves: 2 Total Time: 20 min

Ingredients:

- 4 cups of green cabbage, shredded
- 1/3 cup of macadamia nuts, chopped
- 1 tsp. of vinegar
- 1 tsp. of chili paste (or vegan kimchi paste or sriracha, if preferred)
- 1 Tbsp. of tamari (substitute with liquid aminos, if preferred)
- 2 cloves of garlic, minced
- 1 Tbsp. of sesame oil
- Green onion and sesame seeds to garnish (if preferred)

Instructions:

1. Put the cabbage, vinegar, tamari, chili paste, and sesame oil in a pan at medium-low heat setting.
2. Toss the minced garlic in.
3. Cover the pan. Allow to cook for about 5 minutes or until the cabbage begins to soften.
4. Stir thoroughly to make sure that everything is well combined. Add the nuts.
5. Allow cooking for 5 minutes more or until the nuts begin to soften and absorb some of the liquids.
6. Garnish with onions and sesame seeds. Serve and enjoy!

Kale Pate and Spread

Serves: 10 Total Time: 15 min

Ingredients:

- 1 head of kale (purple, green, or dino), chopped
- 8 pcs. of onions (green part only)
- ½ cup of organic sesame seeds, raw
- 1 Tbsp. of extra-virgin olive oil
- 1 ¼ tsp. of grey sea salt
- 3 Tbsp. of apple cider vinegar

Instructions:

- Heat 1 Tbsp. of olive oil and chopped kale in cast iron pan at low heat setting. Cover and allow to cook until slightly crispy or for about 7 minutes.
- Remove from pan and transfer to a blender or a food processor with an S-type blade.
- Add the rest of the ingredients. Process until a smooth consistency is achieved. Make sure to use the tamper of the blender to push down the ingredients to the blade.
- Spoon contents into a Mason jar. Refrigerate for 4 to 5 days.
- Serve cold!

Crumbly Keto Almond Feta

Serves: 10 Total Time: 12 to 24 hours

Ingredients:

- 1 cup of almonds, soak for 8 hours or more
- 3 Tbsp. of olive oil
- 3 Tbsp. of lemon juice (substitute with white wine vinegar, if preferred)
- 1 clove of garlic

- 4 to 8 Tbsp. of water
- ½ tsp. of salt

Instructions:

1. Remove the skins of the soaked almonds by squeezing. Place them in blender or food processor together with the oil, lemon juice, salt, and garlic. Process the ingredients until you achieve a smooth mass. Add some extra water, if necessary to facilitate the blending process.
2. Place a colander on a small-sized bowl, and then cover with several cheesecloth layers or a clean, thin tea towel. Scoop the pureed almond nut cheese through the colander. Fold the cheesecloth or tea towel around the cheese in a way that you can squeeze it into a ball.
3. Allow it to sit for about 12 to 24 hours under room temperature or until it dries, out and ferments a bit. Skip this step if you prefer to bake the dish right away.
4. Pre-heat the oven at 400° F. Cover a baking sheet or oven rack with parchment paper. Remove the cloth from the cheese. Place the cheese on the parchment paper. Pat the ball a beet if you wish to make it wheel-shaped. Smoothen any uneven patches or cracks.
5. Allow to bake for around 30 minutes or until it has a firm feel, and the rind turns golden brown. Allow to cool down

before refrigerating to make it firmer. When refrigerated, it can last for a few weeks.

6. Best served and enjoyed cold!

Vegan Keto-Style Mozzarella Sticks

Serves: 10 sticks (1 stick/serving) Total Time: 11 min

Ingredients:

- 10 pcs. of hearts of palm
- 2 Tbsp. nutritional yeast
- 2 Tbsp. of lupin flour (replace with soy or chickpea flour, as desired)
- 1 tsp. of dried oregano
- ¼ tsp. of granulated garlic
- 1 pinch of ground black pepper
- 1 pinch of salt
- 1 Tbsp. of olive oil
- 3 Tbsp. of water

Instructions:

1. Pre-heat oven to 375° F. Has a rimmed baking sheet w/ parchment paper lining on hand.
2. Drain hearts of palm.
3. Get a flat dish with wide enough width to fit a whole heart of palm w/ some room. Whisk dry ingredients together. Stir the olive oil and water in. Make sure to stir all lumps out until the batter becomes smooth.
4. Roll each hart of palm around until it is coated in the batter completely. Put the finished palms on a baking tray. Allow to bake for around 20 to 25 minutes or until the coating becomes firm, and golden all over.
5. Best eaten dipped in marinara. Enjoy!

Conclusion

I would like to thank you and congratulate you for transiting my lines from start to finish.

I hope this book was able to help you learn everything you need to know about the healthy vegan keto diet.

The next step is to everything you learned from this book, and enjoy the numerous health benefits that adopting a vegan keto diet can offer.

I wish you the best of luck!

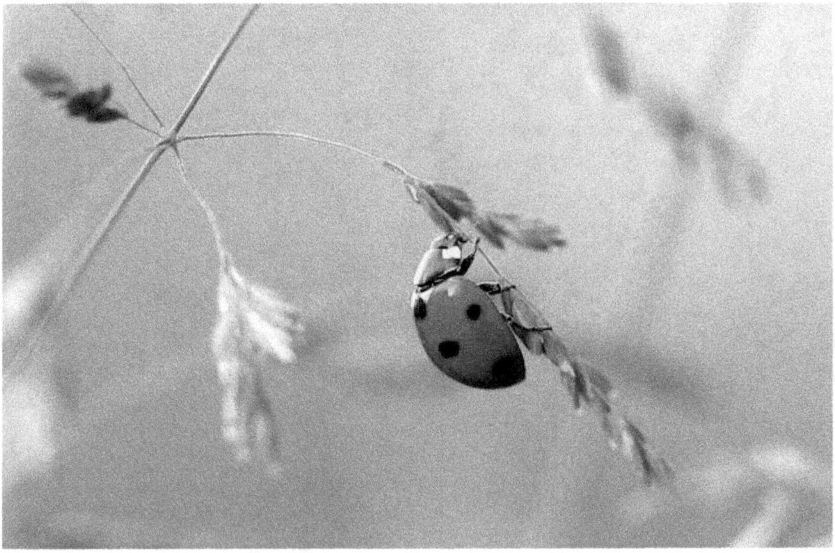

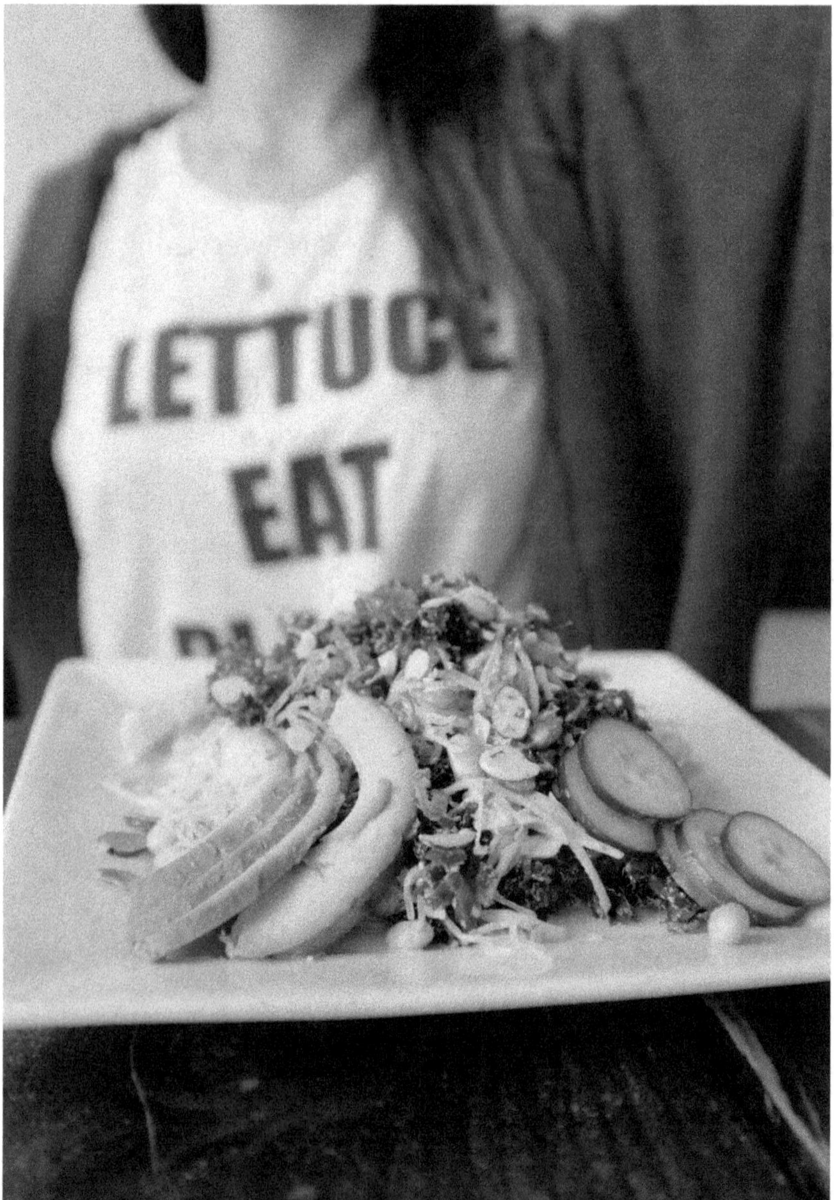
LETTUCE
EAT

CPSIA information can be obtained
at www.ICGtesting.com
Printed in the USA
LVHW021323091120
671125LV00003B/355

9 781801 110082